Schizophrenia
Second Edition

EDITED BY
SOPHIA FRANGOU MSC MRCPSYCH
SENIOR LECTURER

AND

ROBIN M MURRAY MD DSC FRCP FRCPSYCH
PROFESSOR OF PSYCHIATRY
INSTITUTE OF PSYCHIATRY
DE CRESPIGNY PARK
DENMARK HILL
LONDON, UK

MARTIN DUNITZ

Although every effort has been made to ensure that the drug doses and other information are presented accurately in this publication, the ultimate responsibility rests with the prescribing physician. Neither the publishers nor the author can be held responsible for errors or any consequences arising from the use of information contained herein.

First published in the United Kingdom in 2000 by
Martin Dunitz Ltd
The Livery House
7–9 Pratt Street
London NW1 0AE

Tel: +44-(0)20-7482-2202
Fax: +44-(0)20-7267-0159
E-mail: info@mdunitz.globalnet.co.uk
Website: http://www.dunitz.co.uk

Cover illustration by Greg Becker.

A CIP catalogue record for this book is available from the British Library

ISBN 1-85317-920-5

Distributed in the United States by:
Blackwell Science Inc.
Commerce Place, 350 Main Street
Malden MA 02148, USA
Tel: 1-800-215-1000

Distributed in Canada by:
Login Brothers Book Company
324 Salteaux Crescent
Winnipeg, Manitoba R3J 3T2
Canada
Tel: 1-204-224-4068

Distributed in Brazil by:
Ernesto Reichmann Distribuidora de Livros, Ltda
Rua Coronel Marques 335, Tatuape 03440–000
Saō Paulo
Brazil

Composition by Wearset, Boldon, Tyne and Wear
Printed and bound in Italy

Contents

Dedication

This book is dedicated to those who have suffered a psychotic illness in the hope it may contribute to their better care

Clinical features and diagnostic issues

1

Characteristic symptoms

The clinical presentation of schizophrenia varies both
between individuals and within the same individual at
different stages of the illness, but the following are among the
most common features.

Abnormal thoughts

Delusions are false beliefs, based on incorrect inference about
reality, that are inconsistent with patient's educational and
cultural background and are not amenable to reasoning.
Paranoid delusions (persecutory delusions and delusions of
reference) are particularly common. Somatic, religious,
nihilistic or grandiose delusions may also occur, and not
uncommonly patients express complex delusions with
pseudoscientific or pseudophilosophical content.

Persecutory delusions	*Belief that one is harassed or persecuted*
Delusions of reference	*Belief that events, objects or the behaviour of others refer to oneself*
Delusions of control	*Belief that one's thoughts, emotions or movements are controlled by external forces*

Thought process and speech

Disorders of thought process (formal thought disorders) are inferred from abnormalities observed in the spoken and written language of the patient.

Loosening of associations	**The logical associations between the ideas expressed are loose or incomprehensible; when severe, speech becomes incoherent**
Poverty of content of speech	**Speech is sufficient in amount but conveys little information owing to vagueness, stereotypy or repetition**
Thought block	**A sudden interruption in the train of thinking**
Neologisms	**Idiosyncratic words or phrases invented by the patient**

Abnormal perceptions

Hallucinations are sensory perceptions in the absence of external stimuli; auditory hallucinations (especially voices) are by far the most common type of hallucination in schizophrenia. Their content varies, being threatening, insulting, obscene, commanding or helpful. According to their form they are classified as:

Second person	**Voices address the patient directly**
Third person	**Voices discuss the patient in the third person**
Running commentary	**Voices commenting on the patient's actions, referring to him/her in the third person**
Thought echo	**Voices repeat the patient's thoughts**

Visual, tactile, olfactory and gustatory hallucinations can occur but are less common. Occasionally, schizophrenic patients report bizarre sensations in body organs such as burning in the brain or bursting of blood vessels.

Abnormal affect

The most characteristic affective abnormalities in schizophrenia are reduction in the intensity of emotional expression or inappropriate emotional expression.

Blunt or flat affect	**A quantitative abnormality with reduction in emotional intensity and variation**
Inappropriate or incongruous affect	**A qualitative abnormality in which the affective response is incompatible with the ideas or thoughts expressed**

Anhedonia is common even in the absence of any other symptoms of depression, but schizophrenic patients often become depressed. At the onset of illness or during acute exacerbations, patients may experience intense emotions such as terror, anxiety or exhilaration in response to the content of their delusions.

Passivity phenomena

These can take the form of:

Thought broadcasting	**The experience of one's thoughts becoming available to the outside world**
Thought insertion	**The experience of alien thoughts being inserted into one's mind**
Thought withdrawal	**The experience of one's own thoughts being removed from one's mind**
Made feelings	**Feelings are experienced as being imposed by an external agency**
Made actions	**Simple actions or complex behaviour are experienced as being caused by an external force**

Motor abnormalities

Disturbances in motor behaviour were an essential part of the early descriptions of schizophrenia but their grosser manifestations are now less common in Western cultures. Either quantitative or qualitative changes may occur:

Posturing	Voluntary adoption of bizarre or inappropriate positions for prolonged periods; may have some symbolic meaning
Waxy flexibility	Sustaining for a prolonged time the position in which the body or limbs are placed
Negativism	Automatic resistance to instructions or attempts at movement
Echopraxia	Pathological, automatic imitation of another person's movements
Stereotypy	Repeated, purposeless pattern of actions
Catatonic excitement	Intense, purposeless and disorganized activity
Catatonic stupor	Immobility and apparent unawareness of surroundings

Cognitive defects

Schizophrenic patients are usually orientated in time, place and person. However, attention and concentration are often impaired, and memory and learning may be poor. For many years these cognitive deficits were thought to be secondary to factors such as poor motivation and distraction by psychotic symptoms. However, in the past few years neuropsychological deficits have come to be seen as an intrinsic part of schizophrenia; these are discussed in detail in chapter 5.

Lack of volition

Patients, especially in the chronic stages of their illness, show lack of drive or initiative and diminished interest in the outside world.

Lack of insight

The vast majority of patients either lack awareness of their mental condition or have reduced awareness of it. Poor insight is associated with non-compliance with medication, increased severity of psychopathology and frequent hospital admissions.[1]

Schizophrenic symptoms can be seen to represent either an excess or a distortion of normal function (positive symptoms) or a decrease or loss of normal function (negative symptoms).

Positive symptoms
Formal thought disorder
Disorganized behaviour
Inappropriate affect
Delusions
Hallucinations

Negative symptoms
Poverty of thought and speech
Impaired volition
Blunt affect and anhedonia
Social withdrawal

When the segregation of schizophrenic symptoms is examined in chronic patients,[2] three core syndromes emerge (Table 1).

Negative symptoms tend to cluster together as part of a syndrome termed psychomotor poverty. On the other hand, positive symptoms fall into two separate clusters. Delusions and hallucinations frequently coexist in the same patient; this syndrome is termed reality distortion. Disorganized thought, bizarre behaviour and inappropriate affect also tend to group together as a second positive syndrome called disorganization.

Table 1
Clinical syndromes in schizophrenia.

Syndrome	Main symptoms
Psychomotor poverty	Poverty of speech Decreased spontaneous movement Unchanging facial expression Paucity of expressive gesture Lack of affective responsiveness, Lack of vocal inflection
Disorganization	Inappropriate affect Incoherent speech Poverty of content of speech
Reality distortion	Delusions Hallucinations

The clinical phases of schizophrenia

Premorbid and prodromal phases

Social and cognitive deficits in schizophrenic patients can be traced back to childhood. Jones *et al.* (1994)[3] obtained prospective data on 4,746 people born in the UK during one week in 1946 and confirmed the previous (mostly retrospective) reports of subtle motor, linguistic and social dysfunction in children who later develop schizophrenia. The preschizophrenics showed increased deviance with age, and cognitive slippage became progressively more marked in early adolescence (Figure 1).

This premorbid phase merges into a prodromal phase in which actual functional decline may be accompanied by odd ideas, eccentric interests, changes in affect, unusual speech and bizarre perceptual experiences.

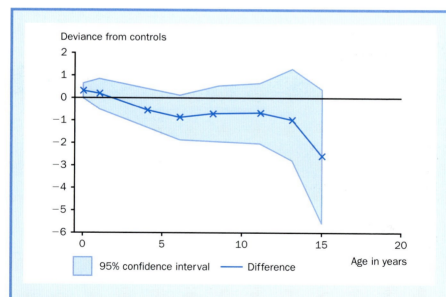

Figure 1
Cumulative developmental deviance from birth to 15 years. the deficit shown by children destined to become schizophrenic increases with age (negative score represents poorer performance by cases). From Jones et al. (1995).[4]

The onset of the prodromal phase is often insidious and gradual and, because the symptoms are non-specific, it is often difficult to draw a line between premorbid personality and the prodromal phase.[5]

Acute phase

In the 1970s, the World Health Organization (WHO) carried out an International Pilot study of Schizophrenia (IPSS) in nine countries in order to determine whether schizophrenia could be reliably diagnosed in all cultures. It could, and the most frequent symptoms of acute schizophrenia found in the IPSS are shown in Table 2.[6]

Course

For much of this century, the course of schizophrenia was considered to be one of continuous deterioration. Today, most clinicians would agree that this extremely pessimistic view is not justified and that there is a great degree of variability in the course:

Table 2
The 10 most frequent symptoms of acute schizophrenia.[6]

Symptom	Frequency (%)
Lack of insight	97
Auditory hallucinations	74
Ideas of reference	70
Suspiciousness	66
Flatness of affect	66
Second person hallucinations	65
Delusional mood	64
Delusions of persecution	64
Thought alienation	52
Thoughts spoken aloud	50

- **Nevertheless, schizophrenia tends to run a prolonged course. Those who recover can experience acute relapses even after years of remission.[7]**

- **The greatest variability in the course of schizophrenia is found in the initial stages. To a large extent, the course appears to be established within the first 5 years following onset.[8,9]**

- **Very few studies have followed schizophrenic patients beyond the middle decades of life. Such studies[7,10] indicate a slight overall trend towards clinical improvement and reduction of positive symptoms with increasing age.**

- **In most cases, schizophrenia seems to follow one of four broad patterns (Figure 2).[9]**

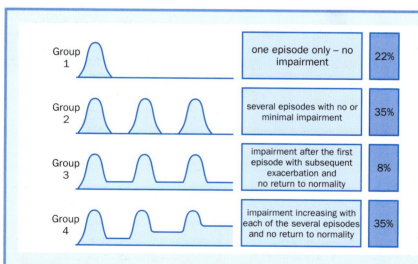

Figure 2
Graded course of illness in first-admission schizophrenic patients as indicated by episodes of illness, symptomatology and social impairment at assessments during 5 years (n = 49). From Shepherd et al. (1989).[9]

Table 3
The outcome of schizophrenia. See Ram et al. (1992)[8] for details of individual studies.

Study	Mean duration of follow-up (yrs)	Number of patients	Good clinical outcome (%)	Poor clinical outcome (%)	Social recovery (%)
Ciompi (1980)	37	289	27	42	39
Bleuler (1978)*	23	208	20	24	51
Bland and Orne (1978)	14	90	26	37	65
Salokangas (1983)	8	161	26	24	69
Shepherd et al. (1989)	5	49	22	35	45

Only 66% of the sample were first admissions.

Outcome and prognostic factors

The outcome of schizophrenia can best be considered along two major dimensions: one is the degree of symptomatic recovery and the other is the level of social functioning. Long-term outcome studies are beset with methodological difficulties but most have reported similar findings. Data from recent first admissions studies are summarized in Table 3.

It can be seen that although clinical and social morbidity tend to be closely associated, social recovery commonly occurs in spite of persistent symptoms. Thus, a substantial proportion of patients, mostly women, show minimal or moderate social impairment despite the continuing presence of schizophrenic symptoms.

Curiously, the IPSS[6] found that outcome appears to be more favourable in developing countries than in developed countries. At 5-year follow up, 45% of schizophrenic patients in developing countries were regarded as clinically recovered and 75% had either no or minimal social morbidity. In developed countries, these figures were 25% and 33%, respectively.[11]

The wide spectrum of outcome in schizophrenia, ranging from recovery to severe disability, undermines the predictive validity of the traditional criteria used in the diagnosis of this disorder. A large body of literature has been devoted to the search for predictors and modifiers of outcome in schizophrenia. Robinson *et al.* (1999)[12] found that, although the majority of patients (87%) recovered from their initial psychotic episode, relapse rates were high, with 81.9% of patients experiencing at least one further episode within 5 years. The risk of relapse was increased five-fold in those patients who discontinued antipsychotic treatment. Poor premorbid function was the most significant predictor of early relapse. Interestingly, clinical features, cognitive function and brain morphological measures were not related to time to relapse. About 8.4% of patients never recovered from their first episode. A similar picture emerges from a Dutch study by Wiersma *et al.* (1998),[13] in which 70% of the patients had at least one relapse within the 5 years after onset and 11% never had a relapse, and from a Japanese study by Ohmori *et al.* (1998) which reported relapse rates of 60% within 5 years of onset.[13] These last two studies also reported that over a 15-year follow up period the rates of relapse appeared to decrease substantially, although only 10–12% of patients were still in remission at the end of the follow-up period.

Although prediction on an individual basis is not possible at present, several factors have been statistically associated with good outcome (Table 4).

Death is the most unfortunate outcome of schizophrenia. The life span of schizophrenics is shortened by 10 years in males and 9 years in females.[13] About 10% of schizophrenics commit suicide.[15–17] The majority of patients

Table 4
Predictors of good outcome.

Sociodemographic
Married
Female

Premorbid adjustment
No previous psychiatric history
No premorbid personality problems
Good social relationships
Good work/educational record

Clinical features
Acute onset
Older at the age of onset
Short episode
Prompt antipsychotic treatment
Continued use of medication
Absence of ventricular enlargement or sulcal widening
Good neuropsychological functioning

---

kill themselves during the active phase of the illness.[16] The presence of comorbid depressive symptoms and previous suicide attempts increase the risk of completed suicide.[16,17] Prominent paranoid features are also associated with increased risk of suicide, while this risk may be reduced in patients with predominately negative symptoms.[17,18]

However, death from other causes is also increased. Accidents are a major contributor as are deaths from cardiovascular disease.[15] The reasons for the latter are unclear: poor living conditions and nutrition, heavy smoking, decreased access to health-care services, and cardiovascular side effects of antipsychotic agents are possible culprits.

Making the diagnosis of schizophrenia

Schizophrenia is a provisional category which may be superseded when we have a better understanding of the psychoses. In the meantime, since no diagnostic tests are available, the history and examination are the only diagnostic tools. Most current diagnostic systems require the presence of clear evidence of psychosis in the absence of affective symptoms (cross-sectional criteria) and a minimum duration of illness (longitudinal criteria). The criteria employed by the two major current classification systems are outlined in Appendix 1.

Differential diagnosis

A large number of neurological conditions can mimic schizophrenia, but these can usually be diagnosed by the presence of their characteristic physical signs or laboratory abnormalities (Table 5). It is important to exclude the possibility of an organic aetiology, especially:

- *in the presence of unusual or atypical features*

- *at the onset of the psychosis or if relapse occurs after long remission*

- *if there is a change in the quality of symptoms*

- *when onset is in childhood or adolescence or in old age*

Symptoms suggestive of schizophrenia can also be seen in a number of other psychiatric disorders.

Drug induced psychosis

Amphetamines, lysergic acid (LSD) and ecstasy can all produce positive symptoms of schizophrenia, while phenylcyclidine (PCP) can also mimic negative symptoms. Drug-induced psychotic episodes are usually short lived and resolve within days of abstinence from the drug. Patients whose drug-associated psychosis lasts for more than 6 months seem to have more clear-cut schizophrenic symptoms, greater familial risk of psychosis, and premorbid personality problems.[19]

Affective disorders

Distinguishing between affective disorders and schizophrenia can be difficult, since affective symptoms, especially depression, are often present in schizophrenia. It may not be possible to distinguish between affective disorders and schizophrenia on the basis of the mental state examination; additional longitudinal information may be necessary. Indeed, an absolute distinction between schizophrenia and mania or depression may be impossible and, in such situations, a trial of treatment for mania or depression may be advisable.

Delusional disorders

Persistent delusional disorders can be differentiated from schizophrenia on the basis of the content of the delusions, which are not bizarre, and the absence of other schizophrenic symptoms.

Table 5
Differential diagnosis of schizophrenia.

Medical conditions	Psychiatric conditions
Epilepsy (especially temporal lobe epilepsy)	Schizophreniform disorder
Central nervous system neoplasm – esp. frontal or limbic	Acute and transient psychotic disorders
Cerebrovascular accidents	Persistent delusional disorders
Central nervous system trauma	Schizotypal disorder
Neurosyphilis	Schizoaffective disorder
Herpes encephalitis	Drug-induced psychosis
Metachromatic leucodystrophy	Mania
Huntington's disease	Psychotic depression
Wilson's disease	Personality disorder
Systemic lupus erythematosus	Factitious disorder

Epidemiological aspects

2

Epidemiological studies of schizophrenia are plagued by variable diagnostic definitions, difficulties in identification of all the cases in a given population and ambiguity about the precise date of onset.

Incidence and prevalence

- *Schizophrenia occurs in all cultures*

- *Incidence is about 2–4 per 10,000 per year[20]*

- *Lifetime risk is about 1%*

Geographic variation

The World Health Organization examined the occurrence of schizophrenia in 10 different countries.[20] The findings are often misquoted as suggesting that the incidence was the same in all countries. However, a more correct interpretation is that the incidence of broadly defined schizophrenia varied by a

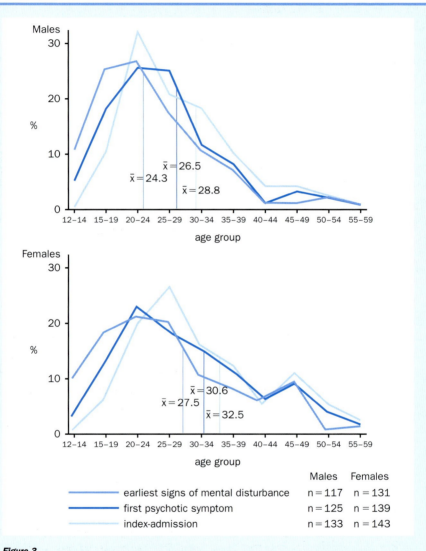

Figure 3
Sex-specific age distribution at different points in time in the early course of schizophrenia (broad definition). From Hafner et al. (1994).[23]

factor of four but the study did not have sufficient statistical power to establish whether or not narrowly defined schizophrenia varied in incidence.

Temporal variation

There is similar controversy over whether the incidence of schizophrenia varies over time. Hare (1988)[21] argues that the incidence rose substantially during the 19th century, and others suggest that the incidence is now declining.[22] However, sceptics consider that this apparent rise and then fall is an artefact of changing policies in the care of the severely mentally ill.

Age and sex

*   Generally, men become schizophrenic about 5 years earlier than women[23]

*   The peak incidence of onset is between 15–25 years in men and between 25–35 years in women[23] (Figure 3).

*   There may be sex differences in total lifetime risk for schizophrenia. Although the IPSS found nearly equal cumulated risks for both sexes[20] up to the age of 54, other studies have reported increased risk strictly defined schizophrenia in men[24]

Social factors

Socioeconomic status

*   **In industrialized countries, there are more schizophrenic patients in the lower socioeconomic classes**

*   **Admission rates for schizophrenia are higher in urban areas than in rural areas, and within urban settings they are higher in the socially disadvantaged areas[25,26]**

Two main hypotheses have been put forward to explain these findings.

Social drift hypothesis

This hypothesis postulates that affected people drift down to lower socioeconomic classes as a consequence of the social and occupational incompetence associated with schizophrenia or its prodromes; most schizophrenic patients lead a very restricted lifestyle and become financially disadvantaged[26–28]

Social causation hypothesis

This hypothesis suggests that stresses related to socioeconomic deprivation are risk-increasing factors for schizophrenia.[29,30] Until recently, conventional wisdom supported the 'social drift' hypothesis and discounted the causative role of urban deprivation. However, both may play a part.

Immigration

Many studies have reported higher incidence and prevalence of schizophrenia in recent immigrants. Much interest has centred on the high rates of schizophrenia among Afro-Caribbean immigrants to Europe.[31–33] The reasons for this are unclear. It is possible that the stress of leaving one's own country and the difficulty of adapting to a new culture act as precipitants in vulnerable people. Most recent studies discount the previously fashionable idea that the increased rates are an artefact of diagnostic bias reflecting cultural intolerance towards deviant behaviour in immigrants.[34]

Fertility and seasonality of birth

- *Fertility rates are reduced among schizophrenic patients by about 25% compared to the general population*[35]

- *In the northern hemisphere, more schizophrenic patients (an excess of about 8%) are born between January and April. The same applies for the months of July to September in the southern hemisphere.*[30] *Some studies suggest that the season-of-birth effect is a consequence of prenatal exposure to maternal winter viral infections.*

Predisposing and precipitating risk factors

3

The aetiology of schizophrenia may be divided into those factors, largely biological, that appear to predispose to the disorder and those factors, largely social, that precipitate the onset or relapse of the disorder.

Predisposing factors

Genetic factors

Genetic contribution to schizophrenia is well established and is supported by family, adoption, and twin studies.[36]

Family studies

The lifetime risk of schizophrenia in relatives of schizophrenic patients increases with increasing genetic proximity to the affected member (Table 6).

The largest and most recent family study is that carried out by Kendler *et al.* (1994) in Roscommon, Ireland.[37] The lifetime risk of schizophrenia in the first-degree relatives of DSM-IIIR schizophrenics was over 10 times that in the relatives of normal controls; schizoaffective disorder, schizotypal

Table 6
The lifetime risk of schizophrenia in the relatives of schizophrenic patients. From Murray and McGuffin (1993).[36]

Relationship	Percentage that are schizophrenic
Parent	5.6
Sibling	10.1
Sibling and one parent affected	16.7
Children of one affected parent	12.8
Children of two affected parents	46.3
Uncles/ aunts/ nephews/nieces	2.8
Grandchildren	3.7
General population	0.86

personality disorder and other non-affective psychotic disorders appeared to share a familial predisposition with schizophrenia.

Sham *et al.* (1994) have largely confirmed these findings in London.[38] Interestingly, the relatives of early-onset probands had a higher risk of schizophrenia than late-onset cases; this study, like several others, also found that the relatives of female schizophrenics had a higher morbid risk than the relatives of male schizophrenics.

Adoption studies[36]

Adoptee studies have found that the rate of schizophrenia in adopted-away offspring of schizophrenics is higher than that in the adopted-away offspring of normal parents.

Adoptee family studies have found that the rate of schizophrenia in the biological relatives of adoptees who become schizophrenic is higher than that in the adoptive relatives.

Cross fostering studies have found that the offspring of normal parents who, by misfortune, are raised by a schizophrenic adoptive parent do not have an increased risk of the disease.

Twin studies[36]

Monozygotic twins are genetically identical, whereas dizygotic twins share, on average, 50% of their genome, like full siblings. Population-based twin studies have estimated heritability to be as high as 83%.[39] Nevertheless, the fact that monozygotic twins show less than 100% concordance provides strong evidence that schizophrenia is not entirely determined by genetic factors.

Models of genetic transmission

Schizophrenia does not follow a mendelian pattern of transmission. Consequently, a variety of genetic models have been proposed to explain the patterns of familial aggregation.

- **The single locus inheritance model proposes that schizophrenia is due to a single gene of major effect with either incomplete penetrance or variable phenotypic expression.**

- **The polygenic or multifactorial model postulates that schizophrenia results from the combined, additive action of multiple genes, acting together with environmental factors; vulnerability to the disorder is normally distributed in the population but only expressed in those people whose liability exceeds a certain threshold.**

Molecular genetic studies[40]

A full understanding of the aetiology of schizophrenia is only likely to come when the predisposing genes and their cellular functions are identified. Much research is therefore under way that is applying molecular genetic techniques to the characterization of susceptibility genes for schizophrenia. Genome-wide searches by linkage analysis have pointed to various 'hot spots' scattered throughout the genome. At the time of writing, some of the most positive findings have been reported for chromosomes 13q, 22q, 6p and 8p. However, these candidate regions encompass many dozens of genes, and knowledge of the precise identity of the culprits is some way off. A number of other regions that have been tentatively identified as containing a susceptibility gene for schizophrenia include chromosomes 15, 10 and 5, and the velocardiofacial syndrome deletion region on chromosome 22q11. Perhaps the most surprising observation from linkage analysis is that many of the linked regions found in schizophrenia families, such as chromosomes 13q and 22q, also show up strongly in families with bipolar affective disorder.

Pregnancy and birth complications

McNeil (1995)[41] has reviewed the world literature on pregnancy and birth complications (PBCs). He concluded that seven out of eight studies that examined original birth records, and nine out of 13 studies that relied on maternal recall, reported more PBCs in schizophrenics than controls; PBCs appear to be associated with early onset and possibly with male sex.

Prematurity, prolonged labour, hypoxia and fetal distress have all been blamed, and it has been suggested that the common pathophysiological mechanism underlying the effect of PBCs is hypoxic or ischaemic neuronal injury.[42] Certainly, fetal hypoxia may lead to periventricular haemorrhages and possibly subsequent ventriculomegaly. Moreover, some brain structures, especially the hippocampus, that have long developmental periods extending into postnatal life are highly susceptible to hypoxic injury. Some studies, but not all, have found a positive relation between PBCs and ventriculomegaly and generalized increase in brain abnormality in offspring of (mostly male) schizophrenic mothers.[43] More recently, reductions in temporal lobe structures have been reported predominantly in schizophrenic patients who had experienced severe PBCs.[44]

On the other hand, since pre-existing neurological abnormalities, such as neural tube defects, are known to cause birth complications, it is possible that PBCs in schizophrenia may reflect, rather than cause, abnormalities in fetal brain development. Some supporting evidence is provided by reports of disproportionately smaller head size at birth in schizophrenics.[42] The cause could be either a defect in the genetic control of neurodevelopment[45] or earlier environmental damage, such as malnutrition or prenatal viral infection.

Prenatal exposure to viral infection

As noted in chapter 2, more schizophrenics are born in the late winter and spring that would be expected. A number of reports have suggested that exposure to influenza epidemics during the second trimester of gestation increase the subsequent risk of schizophrenia.[42] An almost equal number of reports have been negative, and the theory continues to be highly controversial.[42]

Precipitating factors

Biological predisposition, although important, cannot fully account for the development of schizophrenia. Furthermore, the fluctuations in mental state that are seen in the majority of schizophrenic patients are unlikely to be under strict genetic control. Interpersonal, social and cultural factors have been postulated to influence the course of schizophrenia; of these, family interactions and life events have been the most widely studied.

Family interactions

Brown (1959)[46] observed that schizophrenic patients discharged to homes of spouses and parents had more relapses than patients discharged to homes of siblings or to lodgings. Over the ensuing 35 years a large number of studies have examined the quality of the relationship between patients and their relatives. A semi-structured interview, the Camberwell Family Interview, was devised to rate crucial aspects of family interactions; it yields a cumulative index called Expressed Emotion (EE). Family members are rated high on EE if they score highly on critical comments, hostility and overinvolvement.[47]

High EE has proved to be a robust predictor of symptomatic relapse following discharge.[48] Regardless of the severity of symptoms or the behavioural disturbance manifested by patients, those from high EE families appear to relapse more frequently than patients from low EE families. Frequent contact (more than 35 hours a week) with high EE families further increases relapse rates.[49] In contrast, warmth and positive attitude towards patients may act as protective factors.[48]

However, the question arises as to how specific such effects are for schizophrenia. High EE families appear to have a detrimental effect on the outcome of other psychiatric disorders such as anorexia and depression.

Life events

The emphasis on life events in schizophrenia is based on two assumptions: that such events are 'stressful', regardless of whether they are pleasant or unpleasant, and that schizophrenic patients are particularly vulnerable to 'stress'.

Evidence accumulated so far suggests that:

- *compared to other psychiatric groups, schizophrenic patients do not have more life events in the weeks or months before relapse or admission*[50]

- *compared to normal controls, schizophrenic patients may have more life events,*[50] *particularly clustered in the 3 weeks before relapse or admission*

A major problem in the interpretation of these findings is the determination of the direction of causality.[51] Relapse may be a consequence of stressful events but it is also possible that life events may be due to the abnormal behaviour exhibited by patients during the premorbid phase of their illness or the early stages of a psychotic episode. To address this issue, life events can be divided into two groups, depending on whether they are, at least to some extent, under the patient's control (dependent) or not (independent). When this distinction is taken into account, it seems that most of the life events preceding the onset or relapse of schizophrenic symptoms are attributable to the patients' psychiatric condition,[52] although independent life events may also be increased.[53]

Drug Abuse

As noted in chapter 1 (page 11), abuse of some drugs can produce a syndrome that mimics schizophrenia. In addition, there is some evidence that drug abuse can precipitate schizophrenia in those already predisposed.[54,55] Thus, Andreassen *et al.* (1987, 1989)[56,57] found that Swedish conscripts who admitted to frequent cannabis consumption were subsequently more likely than their peers to be admitted to hospital with psychosis over the next 15 years.

Brain abnormalities in schizophrenia

4

Structural brain abnormalities

In vivo studies (neuroimaging)

Structural imaging with computed tomography (CT) and magnetic resonance imaging (MRI) has provided information about morphological and volumetric changes. Brain function has been studied with positron emission tomography (PET), single proton emission tomography (SPET) and functional MRI.

DIFFUSE CHANGES

- *Enlargement of the lateral and third ventricles is the most consistently reported abnormality in schizophrenia (Figure 4). Ventricular volume appears to be increased by about 40% bilaterally, although left-sided increases may be more pronounced[58]*

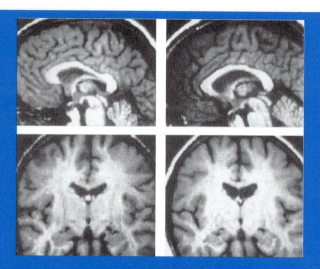

Figure 4
MRI scan of a normal male (left) and a schizophrenic male (right) showing enlargement of the ventricular system.

- In patients with schizophrenia, ventricular enlargement may be associated with impaired performance on neuropsychological tasks and possibly with negative symptoms.[59] Ventricular enlargement may be more prominent in male patients than in female patients[58]

- Whole brain volume reductions have also been consistently reported. These appear to be bilateral and present in both sexes and to occur in 3–4% of patients

REGIONAL CHANGES

- Frontal and temporal lobes
  Post mortem and neuroimaging studies in schizophrenia have repeatedly demonstrated reductions in the volume of the frontal and temporal lobes. Regardless of the methodology employed, these reductions are similar to (or possibly marginally larger than) those reported for whole brain volume[58,60]

- Limbic structures
  The literature regarding abnormalities in the hippocampus–amygdala complex and the parahippocampal gyrus has been less consistent. However, two recent

independent meta-analyses of neuroimaging studies that examined these structures have found that the volume of the hippocampus and amygdala is reduced bilaterally by 4.5–10%.[58,61] The parahippocampal gyrus has received less attention, but the reported volume reductions in this region (9–14%) are probably the largest of any cortical area[58,60]

• **Basal ganglia**
Studies of the basal ganglia have produced contradictory results[62] possibly owing to an increase in basal ganglia volume associated with antipsychotic treatment. Interestingly, these volumetric changes are not seen during treatment with clozapine; indeed, patients switched from typical antipsychotic agents to clozapine show a subsequent decline in basal ganglia volume,[63] which may be relevant to the low potential of clozapine to produce acute extrapyramidal side effects and tardive dyskinesia.

Progression over time

Brain abnormalities are present at the onset of schizophrenia; whether changes in brain morphology are ongoing is highly controversial. The picture emerging from longitudinal studies is rather confusing. Some studies have shown no progression,[64,65] while others have reported changes over time. For example, Gur *et al.* (1998)[66] examined brain morphological changes in first episode schizophrenia patients over a period of 30 months. Total cerebral and ventricular volume remained unchanged, but frontal and temporal lobe volumes showed time-dependent reductions, primarily in the left hemisphere. Surprisingly, this was associated with clinical improvement. DeLisi *et al.* (1998) obtained brain structural data annually

over a 5-year period from 50 patients after their first hospitalization for psychosis.[67] No consistent pattern was found either in the direction of brain morphological changes over time or in the temporal relationship between structural changes and clinical outcome. However, patients with acute onset and complete clinical recovery tended to have the smallest ventricular volume.

Therefore, there appears to be dissociation between clinical severity and degree of brain morphometric deviance. It is likely that changes in brain structure in schizophrenia do not follow a linear pattern but occur in an episodic fashion throughout the course of the disorder. Some support for this view comes from a follow-up study of adolescents with childhood-onset schizophrenia. These patients showed a progressive increase in ventricular volume and a progressive decrease in cortical grey matter volume during adolescence, with frontal and temporal lobes being significantly more affected.[68,69]

Post mortem studies[70]

Most of our current knowledge on the gross morphological changes in schizophrenia comes from neuroimaging studies as described above. The findings of ventricular enlargement and decreased cerebral volume, both diffuse and regional, have also been confirmed by neuropathological studies. The most significant contribution of neuropathology has been in exploring the microscopic correlates of the observed gross abnormalities. The absence of increased gliosis in post mortem schizophrenic brains has been

one of the findings in support of a neurodevelopmental hypothesis for schizophrenia. More recently, it has been suggested that gross volumetric changes in schizophrenic brains may be due not to a loss of neurones but to reduced neuronal and neuropil size.

Functional brain abnormalities
Abnormalities associated with symptom clusters

Liddle *et al.* (1992) claim that each of the three main schizophrenic syndromes described in Chapter 1 is associated with a specific pattern of regional cerebral blood flow changes (rCBF) as measured with PET; rCBF is taken as a proxy for neural activity (Table 7).[71]

Table 7
Clinical syndromes in schizophrenia and associated regional cerebral blood flow (rCBF) patterns.

Syndrome	rCBF pattern
Psychomotor poverty	Decreased rCBF in prefrontal and left parietal cortex Increased rCBF in caudate nuclei
Disorganization	Decreased rCBF in the right ventral prefrontal cortex Increased rCBF in the right anterior cingulate
Reality distortion	Decreased rCBF in the posterior cingulate and left lateral temporal lobe Increased rCBF in the left medial temporal lobe

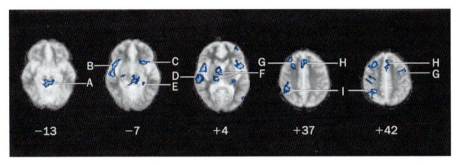

Figure 5
Brain activation during random sampling of hallucinations. Five transverse sections through the brain, at different levels relative to the intercommissural plane (mm). The right side of the brain is shown on the left side of each section. The coloured areas are regions that were activated during auditory hallucinations, with the foci of maximal significance shown in yellow. The main activations (p < 0.0001) were in the right inferior colliculus (A), the right and left insula (B and C), the left parahippocampal gyrus (E), the right STG (D) and right thalamus (F). Activation was also evident in the middle frontal (G), and anterior cingulate gyri (H), and in the right inferior and superior parietal lobule (I).

Certainly, the association between decreased frontal activity and negative symptoms, which constitute the psychomotor poverty syndrome, has been consistently reported regardless of the imaging technique or medication status of the patients.[62]

Abnormalities associated with individual symptoms

Functional imaging studies have also explored the neural substrate of single schizophrenic symptoms, namely hallucinations and passivity phenomena.

Auditory hallucinations

Shergill *et al.* (1999) have shown that auditory hallucinations are associated with an extensive network of cortical and subcortical areas (Figure 5); there is increased rCBF in the frontal and temporal cortical regions and also right thalamus and inferior colliculus.[72] This pattern of activation is remarkably similar to that seen when healthy volunteers generated inner speech.

However, there are two important differences. During auditory hallucinations, there is lack of activation of the supplementary motor area with increased activation of the hippocampus–parahippocampal gyrus. These areas are respectively involved in monitoring self-generated actions and in detecting mismatch between perceived and expected cognitive activity. Thus, these abnormalities may be related to a lack of awareness that inner speech has been generated, which is thought to be the critical deficit underlying auditory hallucinations

- **relative failure of activation of relevant brain areas during cognitive tasks**

- **deviant patterns of activation.**

Visual hallucinations

Ffytche *et al.* (1998) found that hallucinations of colour, faces, textures and objects were associated with increased activity in the ventral extrastriate visual cortex, which persisted even when patients did not actively hallucinate.[73]

Passivity phenomena

Spence *et al.* (1997) used PET to examine cerebral activation in response to performing a paced joystick movement task in schizophrenic patients experiencing passivity phenomena.[74] Patients showed hyperactivation of the parietal and cingulate cortices, which remitted when the passivity experiences improved. This pattern was not observed in patients without such experiences. These hyperactive regions are critically involved in the interpretation of sensory information; the abnormalities seen may lead to lack of awareness that an internal act has been generated and its misattribution to external causes.

Abnormalities associated with cognitive tasks

Two types of abnormalities have been reported:

Relative failure of activation has been most consistently reported in relation to the frontal lobes (hypofrontality).[75] Activation tasks that have been used to probe frontal lobe function include the Wisconsin Card Sorting test (assessing flexibility in problem solving), the Tower of London test (assessing strategy planning), verbal fluency, the Stroop Task (assessing the ability to suppress inappropriate responses) and the continuous performance test (assessing sustained attention). Functional imaging studies carried out while patients performed such tests have shown failure to activate different regions of the frontal lobe and connected areas.[75]

Deviant patterns of brain activation have been observed in studies examining verbal fluency or flexibility in problem solving in which patients fail to demonstrate the reduction in temporal activity that is found in normal controls when performing the same tasks.[76] Such findings suggest a disruption in frontotemporal activity and have led to the emergence of the concept of functional disconnectivity as a key defect in schizophrenia.

Abnormal neuronal metabolism

Magnetic resonance spectroscopy

Magnetic resonance spectroscopy (MRS) can be used to extract in vivo biochemical information from the brain. The value of this technique lies in the fact that it is the only available in vivo method that allows for the investigation of dynamic processes at neuronal level. The two most commonly used techniques are proton (^{1}H) and 31-phosphorus (^{31}P) MRS.

Several ^{1}H MRS studies of schizophrenia have focused on changes in *N*-acetyl-aspartate (NAA), a neuronal marker, and in the signal from choline-containing compounds (Cho), a marker of neuronal membrane metabolism. The overwhelming majority of studies have reported changes in the above metabolites in chronic schizophrenia patients in their third and fourth decade of life. Even in studies in which newly diagnosed patients were investigated, their mean duration of illness was about 2 years.[77,78] NAA has been found to be reduced in the frontal lobe and medial temporal structures and possibly in the cingulate gyrus.[78–80] This NAA reduction may be more pronounced in the white matter than in the grey matter.[81] The reduction in NAA does not seem to correlate with the duration of illness, nor does it differ between groups of schizophrenic patients at different stages of

the illness.[82,83] Several studies, but not all, have reported increases in the Cho signal in the frontal lobes and hippocampus–amygdala complex but not in the parietal lobes.[79,84–86]

^{31}P MRS studies in schizophrenia have consistently reported decreased levels of phosphomonoesters (PME), which are the building blocks of neuronal membranes.[87–89] At the same time, levels of phosphodiesters (PDE), which are products of neuronal membrane breakdown, are elevated, although possibly only in the early phases of schizophrenia.[87,89,90]

Taken together, the findings from MRS studies suggest that the neuronal population in the brain regions examined remains stable at least until mid-life. However, neuronal cells may be smaller in size or they may have reduced arborization, hence the reduction in NAA. The abnormalities in the Cho, PME and PDE signals suggest that neuronal membrane metabolism, and consequently synaptic function, are abnormal. These abnormalities are most likely to be ongoing but appear to have periodic exacerbations, possibly during the most active phases of the illness.

Neurotransmitter abnormalities

Dopamine

The dopamine hypothesis in its simplest form suggests that functional hyperactivity of the brain dopaminergic system is partially responsible for the development of schizophrenic symptoms. The hypothesis was initially based on the psychotogenic potential of drugs that increase dopamine availability, such as amphetamines, and on the strong correlation between clinical potency and the binding affinity to dopamine D_2 receptors of traditional antipsychotic agents.[91] A number of PET studies of D_2 receptor density have failed to substantiate initial claims of increased D_2 receptor density in the striatum of schizophrenic patients.[92]

Recently, investigation of the dopamine hypothesis has been reinvigorated by the characterization of at least five distinct neuronal dopamine receptors, two D_1-like receptors (termed D_1 and D_5) and three D_2-like receptors (termed D_2, D_3 and D_4).[91] The D4 receptor has a unique limbic distribution and a high affinity for clozapine and other atypical antipsychotic agents.[93] However, no association has been reported so far between the D_4 receptor and either genetic predisposition to schizophrenia or clinical response to antipsychotic agents.[93] The D_3 receptor appears more promising. It has high affinity for both typical and atypical antipsychotic agents and there is mounting evidence for an association between schizophrenia and a particular polymorphism of this receptor (a serine-to-glycine polymorphism at position 9).[93] In addition, homozygosity of this particular polymorphism is more prevalent in good responders to antipsychotic medication, suggesting that this receptor is an important therapeutic target.

Serotonin

At least 14 different subtypes of 5-serotonin (5-HT) receptors have been identified, and some of them may be of importance in schizophrenia. Hallucinogens, such as lysergic acid (LSD) are $5\text{-HT}_{2a/2c}$ agonists. Atypical antipsychotic agents, such as clozapine, olanzapine and risperidone, are potent 5-HT_2 antagonists and have higher affinity for these than for the D_2 receptors.[94] 5-HT_2 receptors are widely distributed in the frontal cortex and have a modulatory effect on dopaminergic neurones.[94]

Several studies exploring this 5-HT and dopamine interaction support the notion that the clinical efficacy of atypical antipsychotic agents in the treatment of schizophrenia may be due to this combination of strong 5-HT_2 and week D_2 receptor affinity.[94] Indeed, there has been much interest in the possibility that an allelic variant of the 5-HT_{2a} receptor gene, allele 2, may be associated with increased genetic risk of schizophrenia,[95] although it appears to be a gene of very small effect. There is some evidence to suggest that certain polymorphisms in the 5-HT$_{2a}$ and 5-HT$_{2c}$ receptor genes may be relevant to clinical response to clozapine.[93] Research also continues in the functional significance of other 5-HT receptors, including 5-HT$_1$, 5-HT$_6$ and 5-HT$_7$, which may also prove relevant to schizophrenia and the action of antipsychotic drugs.[94]

Excitatory amino acids

Glutamate and aspartate are the two main excitatory amino acids found in the central nervous system. They bind to three groups of receptors called kainate receptors, quisqualate receptors and N-methyl-D-aspartic acid (NMDA) receptors according to their main agonists. A link between excitatory amino acids and schizophrenia was first suggested by the action of phenylcyclidine, a potent non-competitive NMDA antagonist, which can induce a syndrome that mimics not only the positive symptoms of schizophrenia but also the negative symptoms of schizophrenia.[95] Post mortem studies of schizophrenic brains have suggested that NMDA and kainate receptors are decreased in temporal lobe structures, such as the hippocampus and the entorhinal cortex, but are increased in the frontal cortex.[95] In keeping with these findings, reduction in messenger ribonucleic acid that encodes for excitatory amino acid receptors has also been reported in limbic structures.[95]

The neuropsychology of schizophrenia

5

Cognitive deficits are a consistent feature of schizophrenia and have been noted since the early descriptions of the disorder.[96] However, it is only in recent years that they have become a focus of detailed research and a possible target for therapeutic intervention.

The pattern of cognitive deficits

In spite of several methodological issues concerning the large number and the variability of the neuropsychological tests employed and differences in patients' clinical characteristics and medication, the pattern of cognitive deficits that emerges appears consistent. In schizophrenia, there are widespread abnormalities affecting nearly every aspect of cognition.[97]

1. General intellectual ability. The Wechsler Adult Intelligence Scale is the most comprehensive instrument for assessing general intellectual ability (intelligent quotient, IQ). About two-thirds of schizophrenic patients show significant impairments in measures of verbal and non-verbal IQ.

2. Memory. Both verbal and non-verbal aspects of memory appear to be affected in schizophrenia, with verbal memory impairment being a relatively more reliable finding.

About one-quarter of schizophrenic patients show impairment in some aspects of memory.

3. Executive function. This refers to a number of processes, including strategy formation, cognitive flexibility, abstract thinking and complex information processing. Several neuropsychological tests are used to assess executive function, with the Wisconsin Card Sorting test being one of the most popular. Schizophrenic patients show significant impairments in all aspects of executive function, with nearly half performing significantly worse than healthy subjects.

4. Motor function. Schizophrenic patients are impaired on tests of manual dexterity and finger oscillation. Although the degree of impairment may reflect, at least in part, extrapyramidal side effects of neuroleptic agents, the presence of motor abnormalities has been noted even in the premorbid stages of the illness.[98,99]

5. Attention. Nearly all neurocognitive tasks engage attentional mechanisms. Several tests, however, are thought to give a preferential assessment of selective and sustained attention and vigilance. The most widely used of these are the digit span, the Continuous Performance test and the Stroop test. The digit span appears to be the least sensitive in discriminating between schizophrenic patients and control subjects, but nearly two-thirds of schizophrenic patients perform significantly worse than healthy controls on the Continuous Performance and the Stroop tests.

6. Language. Substantial impairment in expressive language has been reported in schizophrenia, mostly from tests of vocabulary and word production. Receptive language has been less frequently assessed; the most commonly used assessment is the Token test, in which patients' performance appears significantly impaired. There is some suggestion that word production tests are susceptible to the effects of medication, since the degree of impairment correlates with doses of medication.

The clinical relevance of cognitive deficits

Heinrichs and Zakzanis (1998),[97] following a comprehensive quantitative review of the literature, concluded that most studies used to examine cognitive deficits in schizophrenia included only limited clinical information. Because of the resulting lack of statistical power, they could report only few correlations between measures of cognitive function and clinical variables: higher levels of medications correlated with degree of impairment in expressive language tests and increased number of hospitalizations correlated with executive deficits as measured by the Wisconsin card sorting test.[97] Studies that have specifically examined the relationship of neurocognitive deficits to clinical symptoms have consistently found that clinical improvement is associated with amelioration of some cognitive symptoms, particularly in the domains of sustained and selective attention.[100–102] In fact, attentional function at first presentation may predict response to neuroleptic treatment.[103]

Although neuropsychological measures do not appear to predict clinical course as measured by time to relapse after initial presentation,[104] they may be associated with measures of functional outcome, such as the ability to work or live independently.[105] Indeed, verbal memory, executive function and selective attention appear to predict the level of patients' overall function in the community or their performance on social problem solving and skills acquisition tasks, or both.[105]

The course of cognitive deficits

Kraepelin's use of the term 'dementia praecox' to describe schizophrenia-like syndromes introduced the concept of cognitive decline as an integral part of the schizophrenic process and started a dispute that remains largely unresolved. Some evidence of premorbid deterioration in general intellectual ability comes from studies that examined changes in IQ or academic competence prospectively in community cohorts unselected for mental

illness. Kremen *et al.* (1998) found that significant IQ decline between the ages of 4 years and 7 years predicted adult psychotic symptoms specifically, without increasing the likelihood of other psychiatric symptoms.[106] Similarly, Jones *et al.* (1994) reported a progressive increase in academic deviance in the premorbid phase as people destined to develop schizophrenia approached adolescence.[107]

On the other hand, Russell *et al.* (1997) reviewed childhood IQ measures of 34 patients who had attended a child psychiatry service and compared them to IQ measures of the same patients obtained in adulthood after a mean follow-up period of nearly 20 years.[108] One-third of the sample had a childhood diagnosis of psychosis and the remainders were split evenly between those with a diagnosis of emotional disorder and those with a diagnosis of conduct disorder. The review found no significant change in full IQ, performance IQ or verbal IQ over the 20-year period. Studies of patients with first episode psychosis have confirmed the presence of cognitive dysfunction in multiple domains as described above without evidence of deterioration over follow-up periods of 1–4 years.[100–102] However, prospective assessments of cognitive function performed on older chronic patients suggest that further cognitive decline may occur with ageing. Waddington and Youssef (1996) assessed 41 severely ill patients, who were middle-aged at baseline, over a 10-year period and reported a moderate but ɲgressive deterioration in cognitive functioɲ. Harvey *et al.* (1999) examined geriatric, institutionalized schizophrenic patients over a 30-month period and found that about one-third of the 326 patients in their sample showed evidence of worsening cognitive function.[110]

One interpretation of the above evidence would be that there are two critical periods in the life trajectory of schizophrenia during which cognitive changes may be taking place; one at the premorbid phase: during late adolescence, and another from the fifth decade onwards.

Effect of pharmacological treatment on cognition

- *Typical antipsychotic agents*
  A number of studies have compared the profile of cognitive deficits of drug-free schizophrenic patients to that of patients on typical neuroleptic agents.[111–113] It appears that during acute treatment, typical antipsychotic agents may worsen attention and motor function,[114] whereas after chronic administration, aspects of cognition, such as sustained attention, spatial abilities and some aspects of executive function, may in fact improve.[99,115] However, treatment with high-dose neuroleptic agents or with neuroleptic agents that have significant anticholinergic properties may contribute to the deficits in motor function and memory.[114,116]

- *Atypical antipsychotics*
  The literature on the effects of atypical antipsychotics on cognition is expanding rapidly. Few of the studies published so far have employed a double-blind, randomized design and most have concentrated on the effects of acute or short-term administration. Few studies have comparison groups and when they do these groups are mostly composed of patients on typical antipsychotic agents. Finally, most of the studies have been sponsored by the industry and the possibility of a bias in favour of the atypical antipsychotic agents cannot be ignored. Because of their favourable extrapyramidal profile, most atypical antipsychotic agents appear to improve motor processing and reaction time

- *Clozapine*
  During acute treatment there does not appear to be a significant difference in cognitive function between patients on clozapine and those on typical antipsychotic agents.[117] With more prolonged treatment, the most significant improvement seen

with clozapine is in verbal fluency.[118] Improvements may also be seen in attention and perseveration, with limited impact on measures of other aspects of executive function.[99] No consistent association has been found between cognitive response to clozapine and symptomatic response to clozapine, although a history of clinical response to previous treatment with typical neuroleptic agents appears to predict cognitive improvement on clozapine.[118]

- Risperidone
  Treatment with risperidone may improve some aspects of attention and executive function, such as working memory, but not verbal fluency.[118] Improvements have also been reported in verbal and spatial memory and verbal learning.[99,118] As with clozapine, the degree of symptomatic recovery is not associated with cognitive improvement.[118]

- Olanzapine
  Initial investigations on the effect of olanzapine in schizophrenia suggest that it may produce significant improvements in verbal learning and memory and verbal fluency.[118]

- Quetiapine
  A single small study reported that schizophrenia patients who were changed from typical neuroleptic agents to quetiapine showed improvements in measures of attention.[119]

To date, there are no published reports on the cognitive effects of the other atypical antipsychotic agents.

Drug treatment

6

A huge variety of antipsychotic drugs have been developed over the past 40 years. Although their chemical structure varies widely, they can all be used in the treatment of schizophrenia and other psychoses (i.e. they are antipsychotic in general rather than antischizophrenic in particular).

Typical and atypical antipsychotic agents

The term neuroleptic was introduced by Delay and Deniker (1957)[120] to characterize compounds that

- had an antipsychotic effect that was not due to sedation;

- reduced psychomotor activity; and

- produced parkinsonism in humans and catalepsy in animals.

These neuroleptic compounds, are now also termed 'typical' antipsychotics, to distinguish them from newer 'atypical' antipsychotic drugs.

Table 8
Commonly used typical antipsychotic agents.

Drug	Chemical group	Dose range (mg/day)
Chlorpromazine	Phenothiazine (aliphatic)	25–1000
Thioridazine	Phenothiazine (piperidine)	150–800
Trifluoperazine	Phenothiazine (piperazine)	10–45
Flupentixol	Thioxanthine	6–18
Haloperidol	Butyrophenone	1.5–200
Pimozide	Diphenylbutyl piperidine	2–20

Atypical antipsychotic drugs comprise a varied group of compounds that share a number of characteristics:

- they attempt to cause a preferential reduction in the spontaneous firing of the mesolimbic dopaminergic neurones with little effect on the nigrostriatal neurones;

- have higher 5-HT$_2$ than D$_2$ dopamine receptor affinities;

- they do not produce sustained elevation of prolactin; and

- they have low propensity for catalepsy in animals or extrapyramidal side effects (EPS) in humans.

Typical neuroleptics

Phenothiazines, butyrophenones, thioxanthines and diphenylpiperidines are considered typical antipsychotics. A list of those most commonly used is provided in Table 8. They all show an affinity for the D$_2$ dopamine receptors, which are mostly located in the nigrostriatal and the mesolimbic dopamine pathways. Such typical drugs are more effective in the treatment of the positive symptoms of schizophrenia than the negative symptoms. There is no convincing evidence to suggest that, when optimally used, any one of these drugs is superior to any other in the treatment of schizophrenia. They do, however, vary in their side effect profile; as a rule, the higher the potency, the greater the risk of EPS; the lower the potency, the greater the risk of sedation, hypotension, anticholinergic effects and seizures.

Atypical antipsychotic agents

The most commonly used atypical antipsychotic agents are listed Table 9.

Clozapine

Clozapine is the prototype atypical antipsychotic agent.[121] It was first introduced in 1970 but was soon withdrawn in many countries because of a series of cases of fatal agranulocytosis. It was reintroduced to those countries from 1990 onwards with strict haematological monitoring. The risk of agranulocytosis (1% of treated patients) is dose-independent[122] and is highest in the first year of treatment. In addition, compared to other neuroleptics, clozapine is associated with increased risk of seizures.

Because of these potentially dangerous side effects, clozapine is mainly used in the treatment of patients who have either failed to respond to treatment with standard antipsychotic agents or who have experienced intolerable side effects.

The pharmacological profile of clozapine differs from that of typical antipsychotic agents in many aspects.[123] It has low affinity for D_2 dopamine receptors and high affinity for the D_4 dopamine receptors. In addition, compared with typical drugs, clozapine also has high affinity for a number of serotonin receptors, including 5-HT_2, 5-HT_1 and 5-HT_3 receptors. The reason for clozapine's increased efficacy and low EPS is not clear. Some ascribe it to its combination of low D_2 and high D_4 affinity, others to its high 5HT_2:D_2 ratio.[123]

Table 9
Atypical antipsychotic agents.

Drug	Chemical group	Dose range (mg/day)
Drug	Chemical group	Dose range (mg/day)
Clozapine	Dibenzodiapezine	150–900
Olanzapine	Thienobenzodiazepine	10–20
Risperidone	Benzisoxazole derivative	4–8
Quetiapine	Dibenzothiazepine	300–750
Amisulpride	Benzamide	400–1200
Zotepine	Dibenzothiepine	75–300

Risperidone

Like clozapine, risperidone is a more potent 5-HT_2 antagonist than a D_2 antagonist.[123] Two meta-analyses of clinical trials comparing risperidone to haloperidol suggested that risperidone may be more efficacious in the treatment of positive and negative symptoms and has reduced risk of EPS.[124,125] However, its affinity for D_2 dopamine receptors is higher than that of clozapine and may account for the dose-related EPS[4] that become more pronounced above a dosage of 6 mg/day. Dose-related increases in prolactin levels are also seen and have been associated with sexual dysfunction. Other common side effects include insomnia, headache, nausea and vomiting, somnolence, dizziness and fatigue.[126]

Olanzapine

Olanzapine has a chemical structure that is similar to that of clozapine. It shows high affinity for $5-HT_{2a}$ receptors and a D_2 affinity that is less than that of haloperidol but greater than that of clozapine. It also binds strongly to α_1- and α_2-adrenergic, histaminergic and muscarinic receptors.[127] Clinically, it appears to be as effective as haloperidol in reducing positive symptoms of schizophrenia and may be superior to haloperidol in the treatment of negative symptoms.[127] It appears to be have few EPS and to cause minimal elevation of

prolactin.[122] The most common side effects are sedation and weight gain; others include dizziness, postural hypotension, peripheral oedema, dry mouth and constipation.[127]

Quetiapine

Quetiapine, like clozapine, binds strongly to $5-HT_2$ receptors and has relatively lower D_1 and D_2 affinity. It also exhibits histaminergic and α_1-adrenergic binding with moderate α_2-adrenergic activity. Its clinical efficacy is comparable to that of haloperidol or chlorpromazine in the treatment of both positive and negative symptoms.[128–130] Its propensity to produce EPS appears remarkably low across the dose range.[130] It is not associated with sustained elevation in prolactin levels and consequent endocrine changes. Other common side effects include dizziness, hypotension, somnolence and weight gain.[131]

Amisulpride

Amisulpride binds strongly to D_2 and D_3 but not to D_1 receptors.[132] Its binding profile is highly selective and shows no affinity for serotonergic, α-adrenergic or histaminergic receptors.[133] Its affinity for limbic dopaminergic receptors is three times higher than for the striatal ones.[132] This possibly accounts for the more favourable EPS profile, although a dose-dependent increase of EPS is seen at higher therapeutic doses.[122,134] At low doses, it preferentially blocks presynaptic dopamine autoreceptors, effectively increasing dopamine release; at higher doses, it acts as a postsynaptic dopamine receptor antagonist.[132] At doses of 400–800 mg/day, it is as effective as haloperidol in the treatment of positive symptoms,[135] while it may be superior in the treatment of negative symptoms, even at lower doses.[136]

Ziprasidone

Ziprasidone has the highest $5\text{-}HT_2:D_2$ ratio of all atypical neuroleptic agents. It binds strongly to $5\text{-}HT_{2a}$ and $5\text{-}HT_{1c}$ receptors and has considerable affinity for dopamine D_4 receptors.[137] Its affinity for α_2-adrenergic receptors as well as for histaminergic and muscarinic receptors is very low suggesting that its potential to produce sedation is also low.[138] It also differs from other available neuroleptics in its blocking of noradrenaline reuptake and its $5\text{-}HT_1$ agonist properties. Initial results from clinical trials suggest that ziprasidone has similar efficacy to that of haloperidol in the treatment of positive symptoms and may have additional antidepressant properties.[139,140] It side effect profile appears favourable in terms of EPS and weight gain.[139]

Zotepine

Zotepine has high affinity for D_1, D_2, D_3 and D_4 and $5\text{-}HT_{2a}$ and $5\text{-}HT_{2c}$ receptors.[141] It also binds to α_1-adrenergic and H_1 histaminergic receptors.[141] The efficacy of zotepine in the treatment of positive symptoms appears to be similar to that of haloperidol, but it may be superior in treating negative symptoms.[142,143] Zotepine is a sedative antipsychotic agent[144] with significant cardiovascular side effects, particularly postural hypotension and prolongation of the QT interval.[141] It produces electroencephalographic abnormalities and has been associated with an increased, dose-dependent risk of seizures.[145]

Side effects

Antipsychotic agents produce extensive side effects that are often distressing to patients and occasionally dangerous.

Central nervous system effects
Sedation

Sedation is frequently seen early in treatment. It is mainly mediated through D_2, H_1 and α_1-adrenergic receptor antagonism.

Treatment

Reducing the dose or giving the medication in a single bed-time dose may reduce daytime sedation.

Extrapyramidal side effects

EPS include muscle spasms, tremor, dystonia, akathisia and drug-induced parkinsonism. They result form blockade of D_2 receptors in the nigrostriatal pathway. EPS can occur with any antipsychotic agents but are especially common with high-potency, traditional neuroleptic agents. All atypical antipsychotic agents have a lower propensity to produce EPS than traditional neuroleptic agents. For clozapine, olanzapine and quetiapine, the liability to produce EPS appears to be independent of dose within their therapeutic range.[122] This may not be the case with risperidone and amisulpride. At doses less than 8 mg/day, fewer EPS are seen with risperidone than with typical neuroleptics, but this is not the case with higher doses.[146,147] Although there appears to be a dose-related increase in EPS with amisulpride, the overall liability to produce EPS is low across its entire therapeutic range.[148]

Treatment

Anticholinergic drugs such as procyclidine and orphenadrine can alleviate EPS. In acute dystonia they can be given intramuscularly and may reverse the symptoms in minutes. Maintenance anticholinergic treatment is useful in drug-induced parkinsonism, but the need should be regularly reviewed. Anticholinergic drugs are least effective in the treatment of akathisia; treatment options include lowering the dose, changing to an antipsychotic agent with a low EPS propensity or using a β-blocker.

Tardive dyskinesia

Spontaneous dyskinesias have been reported in schizophrenia but their incidence is much less common than that of neuroleptic-induced tardive dyskinesia (TD).[149] About 5% of schizophrenic patients will develop TD for each year of continuing medication. Two main types of movements are included under the heading of TD.

- *stereotypies*

- *dystonia*

Stereotypies most commonly involve the orofacial region and can take the form of repetitive chewing-like movements, grimacing, lip-smacking, lip-licking or lip-pursing, lateral tongue movements or tongue protrusion, jaw deviation and blowing movements. Stereotypies can also develop in any part of the body and may be quite complex; patients may cross and uncross their legs, wave their hands or feet, march in place or shift their weight from one leg to another.

Dystonic movements of the cranial and cervical muscles are common. They can include tonic jaw deviation, torticollis, retrocollis, anterocollis and laterocollis. When the truncal muscles are involved, severe scoliosis and posturing may result.

TD most frequently develops during treatment with neuroleptic agents but it can also appear within 6 months of stopping them. Age is the most clearly identified risk factor, with a three-fold increase in the risk of TD in patients over the age of 40 years. Development of EPS early in treatment and pre-existing organic brain disease also appear to increase the risk of TD. Women and patients with affective symptoms may also be at increased risk, but the evidence is not very convincing. The group of neuroleptic agents used does not seem to affect the risk for TD with the exception of atypical antipsychotic agents such as clozapine and possibly risperidone and olanzapine, which may have low propensity for TD.[22]

The pathogenic mechanism of TD has not been fully elucidated. It may involve increased catecholaminergic (both dopaminergic and noradrenergic) activity and reduced GABAergic and cholinergic activity in the pathways that connect the substantia nigra and basal ganglia with the cortex and the thalamic and subthalamic nuclei.

Treatment

Discontinuation of neuroleptic treatment may lead to alleviation of TD, but this is not always possible in patients with severe psychosis. Paradoxically, stopping the neuroleptic agent may exacerbate the movements. Atypical antipsychotic agents, particularly clozapine, have been used in the treatment of TD with beneficial effects. Anticholinergic medication (e.g. benztropine) and GABA receptor agonists such as clonazepam may ameliorate tardive dystonia but have limited effect on dyskinesias. Treatment with dopamine-depleting drugs such as TBZ may be more helpful for the latter.

Seizures

Antipsychotics lower the seizure threshold. Patients receiving low-potency traditional antipsychotic agents or clozapine are more vulnerable, especially if there is a history of seizures.

Treatment

The prophylactic use of anticonvulsants has been suggested for patients receiving moderate-to-high doses of clozapine (>600 mg/day).

Anticholinergic effects

Anticholinergic effects, including dry mouth, blurred vision, urinary hesitancy or retention, constipation, inhibition of ejaculation and cutaneous flushing, are commonly seen early in treatment.

Treatment

In most cases, specific treatment is not necessary since some degree of tolerance almost always develops. If symptoms persist and are particularly distressing, switching to a high potency neuroleptic may be advisable.

Cardiovascular effects

ECG changes (especially widening of the QRS complex and flattening of the T wave), tachycardia and postural hypotension are commonly seen with treatment with antipsychotic agents. These effects are usually benign but can prove dangerous in patients receiving high-dose therapy, in those with co-existing cardiac disease and in the elderly.[122] Recently, there has been considerable debate about the clinical significance of QT prolongation, particularly the possibility that it may be associated with potentially fatal ventricular arrhythmia. All classes of typical neuroleptic agents seem to prolong the QT interval. Pimozide has been associated with sudden death, and it should only be used with

regular EEG monitoring. Among the atypical antipsychotic agents, QT prolongation has been reported with sertindole, which has seen been withdrawn. The reported increase in the QT interval is small with other atypical antipsychotic agents.[122]

Treatment

Treatment with antipsychotic agents should be closely monitored in patients who are on concomitant medication that may affect the QT interval or who have medical conditions associated with cardiac disease or electrolyte disturbances. ECG monitoring is recommended and antipsychotic treatment should be discontinued if the QT interval is longer than 520 ms.

Endocrine effects

Antipsychotic agents increase serum prolactin because they block the inhibitory effect of dopamine on prolactin release from the pituitary stand. This causes reduced release of luteinizing hormone and follicular-stimulating hormone and, in men, reduced testosterone production. In women, symptoms may include menstrual irregularities or amenorrhoea, galactorrhoea and breast enlargement; in men, impotence and gynaecomastia may occur. Patients may be distressed but too embarrassed to complain. Atypical antipsychotic agents are less prone to produce sustained prolactin elevation, with the exception of risperidone and amisulpride, for which dose-related hyperprolactinaemia has been reported.

Treatment

These effects are reversible. The available treatment options are dose reduction or discontinuation or change to an atypical antipsychotic agent.

Skin and eye effects

The most common allergic skin reactions to antipsychotic agents include maculopapular rash, periorbital swelling and urticaria. Chlorpromazine is associated with phototoxic skin reactions resembling sunburns. Continuous use of chlorpromazine or thioridazine for more than 3 years may lead to pigmentary changes in the exposed areas of the skin as well as granular deposits in the cornea and lens. High-dose thioridazine is associated with retinitis pigmentosa with impairment of vision and should therefore be avoided.

Treatment

To avoid phototoxic reactions, patients should be advised to avoid direct sunlight and to use sun blockers. Skin discoloration and granular deposits are reversible on discontinuation of treatment.

Haematological side effects

Benign leucopenia may occur in one in 10 patients receiving antipsychotic agents. Agranulocytosis, a potentially fatal side effect, occurs in about 0.005% of patients treated with typical neuroleptics and in about 1% of patients on clozapine.[122] So far, there have been no reports of agranulocytosis or other clinically significant haematological side effects occurring with risperidone, amisulpride or quetiapine,[122] but there has been one reported case of olanzapine-induced agranulocytosis.[150] Typical antipsychotic agents appear to produce direct bone marrow suppression, while the haematological effects of clozapine are mediated through immunological mechanisms.[122] The risk may be dose-related for typical neuroleptic agents and appears to be dose-independent for clozapine. The elderly, women and patients with a low pre-treatment neutrophil count may be at increased risk.[122]

Treatment

Agranulocytosis should be suspected when patients present with symptoms of infection together with symptoms of bone marrow suppression, particularly in the first 3 months after initiation of treatment. It is usually reversible. Antipsychotic medication should be discontinued and the patient should receive medical treatment.

Hepatic effects

Many antipsychotic agents, including atypical ones, cause minor abnormalities of liver function tests. These are rarely of significance but jaundice is occasionally seen in patients treated with chlorpromazine; it usually presents in the first month of treatment.

Neuroleptic malignant syndrome

Neuroleptic malignant syndrome (NMS) is a rare but potentially lethal complication of antipsychotic treatment; the mortality rate has been estimated to be as high as 20%. It is an idiosyncratic reaction that can occur with any antipsychotic agent, independent of dose and duration of treatment. NMS has been reported with clozapine and risperidone but not, so far, with olanzapine or quetiapine.[22] Patients present with muscular rigidity and worsening of pre-existing extrapyramidal symptoms. Autonomic instability is always present, with tachycardia and hypotension, hypertension or wide swings in blood pressure. Hyperthermia is also seen with temperatures over $41°C$ being common. The patient may be stuporose or delirious or may present with fluctuations in the level of consciousness. Drooling and dysphagia may also be present. Death may result from cardiovascular collapse, renal failure (caused by myoglobinuria following myonecrosis), respiratory failure, pulmonary emboli or aspiration pneumonia.

There are no specific laboratory tests for NMS, but high levels of creatine phosphokinase and aldolase in conjunction with the clinical picture are very suggestive. Liver enzymes may also be elevated.

Treatment

NMS is a medical emergency. Early recognition and intervention are important to prevent mortality. Neuroleptic agents should be discontinued and the patient should be admitted to a medical ward for rehydration, temperature control and monitoring of his or her vital signs and renal function. Bromocriptine enhances dopaminergic activity and dantrolene promotes muscular relaxation and may facilitate recovery.

Weight gain

Weight gain is a common side effect of all antipsychotic agents.[151] It mostly occurs early in treatment and in most patients it stabilizes after 1–2 years of treatment. The average weight gain seen with prolonged treatment is about 10 kg.[151] The most likely mechanisms involved are changed metabolism, particularly the balance between carbohydrate and fat oxidation, and serotonergic blockade, which leads to increased appetite.[151] Weight gain is often ignored by psychiatrists, although it is associated with increased non-compliance and may compromise patients' general health.

Pharmacological treatment strategies

7

Acute treatment

It is important that treatment should begin as soon as possible once the diagnosis is established, since delays in the initiation of treatment may affect outcome. The longer that patients have been psychotic before starting treatment the longer it takes for their symptoms to improve and the level of remission may be compromised.[152] In addition, duration of illness before starting neuroleptic medication may be one of the most important determinants of future relapse.[153]

Which antipsychotic agent?

For the past 40 years, typical antipsychotic agents have been the first-line treatment of schizophrenia. Because they have comparable efficacy, the decision concerning their use is made on empirical grounds and depends on the clinician's preferences, the symptoms to be targeted and the side effect profile of the drug. With the introduction of atypical antipsychotic agents, a re-evaluation of treatment strategies in schizophrenia has begun. Guidelines for the selection and use of all antipsychotic agents are gradually evolving as evidence from clinical trials and the use in practice of atypical antipsychotic agents is accumulating.

Recent evidence suggests that the acute treatment of a first episode schizophrenia may require different pharmacological approaches from that of acute episodes in chronic schizophrenia, and these are therefore considered separately.

Treating first episode patients

Patients with a first episode of schizophrenia may be more responsive to pharmacological treatment, be it with typical or atypical neuroleptics.[154] Lieberman *et al.* (1993)[155] reported rate of recovery of nearly 80% in first episode patients treated with typical antipsychotic agents. In this patient group, low doses of antipsychotic agents (2–6 mg of haloperidol equivalents) are effective, possibly more so than higher doses.[156]

It is not clear whether atypical antipsychotic agents have any advantage over typical neuroleptic agents in the treatment of first episode patients in terms of their efficacy in reducing positive and negative symptoms. Initial data from industry-sponsored studies suggest that the efficacy of risperidone in this patient group may be comparable to that of low-dose haloperidol,[154] while higher responses may be seen with olanzapine.[157]

However, there is little doubt that first episode patients are more sensitive to extrapyramidal effects, with approximately 80% experiencing

such side effects when treated with typical neuroleptics.[154,155] Their prevalence is significantly lower in first episode patients treated with risperidone or olanzapine.[154,157] In this respect, the risk–benefit profile of atypical antipsychotic agents is superior to that of typical neuroleptic agents.

Treating acute exacerbations in chronic patients

The efficacy of atypical antipsychotic agents has been studied more extensively in the treatment of acute relapse in chronic schizophrenia. In nearly all studies, atypical antipsychotic agents have been compared to haloperidol as the standard typical neuroleptic agent. As mentioned in Chapter 6, atypical antipsychotic agents as a group appear to have similar efficacy to haloperidol in the treatment of positive symptoms, may be better at reducing negative symptoms and have a more favourable profile of extrapyramidal side effects.

Studies comparing atypical antipsychotic agents to each other are just beginning and at present there is little evidence to advise clinical practice. In a 28-week, double-blind study comparing treatment response to olanzapine versus risperidone in a sample of 339 patients with schizophrenia and other psychotic disorders, both drugs were found to be effective in reducing psychopathology.[158]

What is an adequate drug trial?

Duration

Although patients vary in their response to antipsychotic agents, most will show some improvement by 2–6 weeks.[159] Different symptoms remit over different periods. The sedative effect of some antipsychotic agents may reduce agitation, hostility and aggression within the first few days of treatment whereas measurable changes in the core psychotic features usually take longer.[160]

Dose

If there is little or no improvement after about 4–6 weeks of treatment with the same antipsychotic agent, it is advisable to continue it for a further 2–4 weeks at a slightly higher dose.[159] It is common for patients who fail to respond to conventional doses of neuroleptic agents to be treated with increasing amounts of medication and for the type of drug to be changed quite frequently. This practice has been recently called into question following studies that have looked at clinical response and receptor occupancy in patients treated with different antipsychotic agents and at different doses. A meta-analysis of 22 randomized controlled trials involving 1638 subjects treated with a range of doses (25–39000 mg of chlorpromazine equivalents, CPZE) has shown that doses higher that 375 mg CPZE confer no additional therapeutic benefit but are associated

with higher rates of side effects.[161] Conversely, doses below 165 mg CPZE seems to be subtherapeutic.[161]

At present, there is little information as to whether prescribing higher doses of atypical antipsychotic agents confers any clinical advantage, although this seems unlikely judging from data that are available on risperidone and olanzapine. Previous studies on a number of typical neuroleptic agents established that doses producing about 80% occupancy of D_2 dopamine receptors were sufficient for antipsychotic efficacy.[162] Nyberg *et al.* (1999)[163] showed that risperidone at a daily dose of 6 mg produced over 80% occupancy of D_2 and 5-HT$_{2a}$ receptors. Even at daily doses of 5 mg, olanzapine produces over 90% occupancy of 5-HT$_2$ receptors, while D_2 receptor occupancy increased with dose.[164] Within the usual dose range of 5–20 mg/day, olanzapine showed 43–80% occupancy of D_2 receptors, while daily doses of 30–40 mg were associated with a small increase in D_2 receptor occupancy, up to 83–88%.[164] From a clinical perspective, analysis of data combined from a number of double-blind studies of patients treated with a range of doses of risperidone have shown that maximum clinical efficacy can be achieved with daily doses of 4–8 mg.[165] Finally, a study of high-dose olanzapine in poor treatment responders showed that only 5% showed any additional improvement.[166]

What is the role of supplemental medication?

There is considerable evidence that adjunctive use of lithium or benzodiazepines may be of some benefit.[159] Psychotic patients with affective symptoms seem to respond to lithium supplementation while benzodiazepines are useful in patients with prominent anxiety or agitation.

Maintenance treatment

Is it necessary? As discussed in Chapter 1, about 20% of patients with schizophrenia do not relapse if treatment is stopped after their initial episode. Unfortunately, at present, it is not possible to identify these patients in advance. In general, about 80% of patients with schizophrenia will experience more than one episodes.[160,167,168] The risk of relapse is about five times higher upon discontinuation of treatment.[167] Based on these probabilistic grounds, maintenance treatment is advisable for almost all schizophrenic patients.

How long should patients stay on maintenance treatment?

There is no point in the course of schizophrenia beyond which the risk of relapse is negligible.[160] Even patients who have been stable for several years run a substantial risk of relapse following withdrawal of medication.[168]

The decision to stop maintenance treatment is therefore a difficult one and needs to be made by the clinician and the patient together. The variables to be considered are:

- **The mental state of the patient at the time**

- **The number and frequency of previous relapses**

- **The risks associated with relapse (with emphasis on dangerous or suicidal behaviour exhibited by the patient during previous acute episodes)**

- **The degree of disruption to the patient's life caused by a further relapse**

- **The level of side effects experienced by the patient and the extend to which they hinder daily living**

- **The presence of an adequate supportive social network**

In any case, stopping medication should not be regarded as an 'either–or' decision. Rather, one should slowly decrease the level of medication over a period of months while monitoring the patient closely for any signs of relapse.

Continuous or intermittent treatment?

The aim of any maintenance treatment strategy is to minimize the risk of tardive dyskinesia (TD) and other side effects while still protecting patients from relapse. Because the atypical neuroleptic agents have been only recently introduced, there is little information with regard to their role in the maintenance phase of treatment. Existing evidence suggests that intermittent treatment is not effective in reducing relapse rates and does not have any advantages in terms of reduced rates of TD or social disability.[169] There are two possible effective strategies:

- **continuous treatment**

- **early initiation of treatment during the prodromal phase of a relapse for those patients who refuse to take medication when in remission but who agree to regular psychiatric monitoring.[169]**

Within this framework, it would appear that new atypical antipsychotic agents may have a better risk–benefit profile as maintenance medication than typical neuroleptic agents do because of their reduced potential to produce TD and other side effects. Tran *et al.* (1998)[170] examined pooled data from three double-blind studies that compared the efficacy of haloperidol and olanzapine during 1 year of maintenance treatment in patients who had responded to these drugs during the preceding acute relapse. The relapse incidents were similar in the two groups (14% for olanzapine and 19% for haloperidol) with a possible advantage of olanzapine in delaying relapse. However, patients on haloperidol were three times more likely to develop TD.[171] The efficacy and safety of risperidone during 1 year of maintenance treatment was examined by Moller *et al.* (1998) in a multicentre open label study.[172] The relapse rate observed was 14% and, although the rates of TD were not reported, there was a time-dependent improvement in rates of extrapyramidal side effects. Finally, Speller *et al.* (1997)[173] compared the clinical efficacy of amisulpride and low-dose haloperidol over a period of 1 year in a sample of chronic patients. They reported that 18% of amisulpride-treated patients and a similar proportion of haloperidol-treated patients had a psychotic exacerbation during the study period. Patients on amisulpride showed improvement in affective flattening and avolition, whereas no significant differences were seen in the rating of positive symptoms. There was no difference in the rates of TD in the two groups at baseline or at study completion.

Oral or depot medication?

Maintenance medication can be given orally or by the intramuscular injection of long-acting formulations of neuroleptic agents (depot).[174] Injectable preparations are currently available only for traditional antipsychotic agents. There are several advantages of depot neuroleptic agents, including improved bioavailability and enhanced compliance.

However, there are important disadvantages as well. Should side effects develop, they can persist for longer, even if the medication is withdrawn, because it usually takes several months for drug plasma levels to decline. Depots are an invasive therapy that carries the risk of tissue damage at the injection site. Many patients find the experience of being regularly injected unpleasant and demeaning. Until now, depot administration has been an efficient strategy for patients whose compliance is doubtful, often a consequence of the development of side effects (see Compliance, pages 57–59). Newer antipsychotic agents have an improved side effects profile and are therefore likely to confer better compliance, reducing the need for depot neuroleptics. However, at present no studies have compared the cost-effectiveness and benefits–risk ratio of oral atypical antipsychotic agents and injectable formulations of typical neuroleptic agents.

How high a dose?

The dosage schedule of any antipsychotic medication in maintenance treatment should aim to balance the risk of relapse against the risk of side effects. In principle, the lowest effective dose needed to prevent relapse should be used for each patient. Studies that have compared different dosing schedules of typical neuroleptics in maintenance treatment in schizophrenia used depot formulations to avoid the problem of covert non-compliance. Generally, doses less than 25 mg fluphenazine fortnightly, 40 mg flupenthixol fortnightly or 25 mg haloperidol monthly result in higher relapse rates.[175] Studies that have examined the efficacy of olanzapine and risperidone in maintenance treatment have found that the average daily dose during this period was within the range used for acute treatment.[170,172]

Drug-resistant schizophrenia

About 30% of schizophrenic patients are poor responders.[176] However, treatment response is not an 'all or nothing' phenomenon and is better understood as a continuum. Some patients make a full recovery on antipsychotic treatment, others continue to present with persistent symptoms and functional impairment, while the majority of patients show intermediate responses with improvement in some areas of functioning but not in all.

In the assessment of treatment resistance the following variables need to be considered.

TREATMENT VARIABLES

- *Covert non-compliance*
  It is important not to confuse treatment resistance with treatment refusal. If non-compliance is suspected, steps should be taken to address this problem before any other strategies are considered (see Compliance, pages 57–59)

- *Drug bioavailability*

- *Therapeutic window*
  Although there are wide individual variations in the plasma levels of antipsychotic agents, the existence of a therapeutic window has been shown for a number of antipsychotic agents; some patients may improve if their medication is reduced.[159]

- *Previous treatment history*
  Sustained periods of active psychosis, if poorly treated or not treated, impair patients' response to subsequent treatment

ILLNESS RELATED VARIABLES

- *Comorbidity*
  Schizophrenic patients who abuse alcohol or drugs or have abnormal premorbid personalities are usually poor responders

- *Early onset*
  An early onset of psychosis (in the adolescent years) is usually an indication of the severity of the illness and of poor therapeutic response

- *The presence of ventricular and sulcal enlargement predicts poor treatment outcome.*

Management

Clozapine

At present, clozapine is the most effective antipsychotic agent available for patients who are poor responders to standard antipsychotic treatment. Between 30 and 60% of such patients will respond to clozapine, and improvement can be detected for up to 1 year.[177,178] This improvement may be greater for negative symptoms and delusions than for hallucinations and thought disorder. Clozapine produces few if any acute extrapyramidal side effects (EPS) and is therefore also helpful for patients who cannot tolerate the EPS produced at standard doses of traditional antipsychotics. In fact, a history of sensitivity to acute EPS or TD is a predictor of good response to clozapine.[177]

As with the traditional neuroleptic agents, treatment response to clozapine may be reduced in patients with early onset of schizophrenia, structural brain abnormalities or prolonged periods of untreated psychosis.[177] A rather unexpected observation is that, although female patients with schizophrenia generally respond better to antipsychotic agents, female treatment-resistant patients seem to do less well on clozapine than male treatment-resistant patients.[177]

Other atypical antipsychotic agents

Apart from a few case reports, systematic data on the efficacy of other atypical antipsychotics in treatment-refractory patients are available only for risperidone and olanzapine. It should be pointed out that the available studies are industry-sponsored and that the authors' own clinical experience suggests that clozapine remains the drug of choice in treatment-resistant schizophrenia.

Risperidone

Three studies have compared the efficacy of risperidone in treatment-resistant

schizophrenia to that of clozapine. Two double-blind studies, one lasting 6 weeks and one lasting 8 weeks, reported similar efficacy for the two drugs in reducing total symptoms[179,180] although clozapine may be marginally superior.[179]

A longer open label study, which lasted 12 weeks, also found that both drugs produced significant and similar improvement in overall psychopathology.[181] Patients on risperidone improved significantly at the beginning of the study and remained stable afterwards. Clinical improvement for patients on clozapine increased over time, suggesting that clozapine may be substantially superior to risperidone if the period of observation is longer.[181]

Olanzapine

An open 6-week study of olanzapine in treatment-resistant schizophrenia reported improvement in positive and negative symptoms over time in a group of 25 patients, with nine patients (36%) achieving *a priori* criteria for treatment response.[182] Breier and Hamilton (1999) compared the clinical efficacy of olanzapine to haloperidol in a subsample of treatment-resistant patients from a larger double-blind trial.[183] Since the parent trial had not been designed to address this issue, this study retrospectively defined as treatment resistant those patients who had failed to respond to at least one neuroleptic over a period of at least 8 weeks and had enduring symptoms. The analysis did not reveal significant differences between the two drugs other than a small to moderate advantage for olanzapine in improving negative and depressive symptoms. Finally, Conley *et al.* (1998) found olanzapine to have similar efficacy to that of chlorpromazine in treatment-resistant schizophrenia, with both drugs producing small to modest improvements in measures of psychopathology.[184]

Adjunctive treatment

A number of studies suggest that the addition of risperidone[185] or sulpiride[186] to clozapine may be a safe and effective approach for the treatment of patients with partial response to clozapine. The addition of benzodiazepines or electroconvulsive therapy to antipsychotic treatment appears to confer some, albeit short-lived, benefits.[187]

Compliance

Compliance is the degree to which patients adhere to a given treatment plan. It is best understood in dimensional terms rather than categorical terms, with some patients being fully compliant with medication, some only partially compliant and some not compliant at all. In schizophrenia, it is estimated that up to 50% of out-patients and 20% of in-patients are not compliant with prescribed medication.[188] This has important clinical and financial implications because non-compliance is associated with high rates of relapse and hospitalization.

The multitude and variety of the variables influencing non-compliance are outlined below and reveal the complexity of the problem.

Demographic variables

Non-compliance is increased in young and elderly patients, in males and in members of ethnic minority groups.[189]

ILLNESS-RELATED VARIABLES

- *Symptomatology*
  Non-compliance may be increased in patients with high levels of positive symptoms, especially grandiose or persecutory delusions and disorganization[188]

- *Refusal to admit illness*
  Lack of insight impairs both compliance with medication and the patient's overall engagement with the psychiatric services[189]

- *Comorbidity*
  Alcohol abuse and substance abuse in schizophrenic patients is associated with non-compliance. Generally, such patients have more severe and persistent psychopathology and a more chaotic life style[188]

SOCIAL AND PERSONAL ATTITUDES

- *Prejudices against treating mental disorders with drugs[189]*

- *Stigma associated with mental illness[189]*

IATROGENIC VARIABLES

- *Underestimation of non-compliance*
  Treating physicians often fail to monitor and reinforce patients' reliability in the management of their medication

- *Lack of information*
  Patients and their carers are often given inadequate information about the diagnosis and the rational for medication. This often leads to dissatisfaction with the quality of care offered, which undermines willingness to follow treatment recommendations

- *Failure to recognize and treat side effects*
  Prophylactic administration of anticholinergic agents, especially on initiation of treatment, may prevent dystonic reactions, which can be distressing and frightening for patients[189]

- *Inconsistency in diagnosis and treatment*
  Patients and carers are often aware of professional disagreements about the diagnosis and treatment of schizophrenia: these can undermine their confidence in a recommended treatment plan[189]

DRUG-RELATED VARIABLES[189]

* Side effects
  Extrapyramidal side effects, particularly akathisia, sexual dysfunction and weight gain, are the most common predictors of non-compliance

* Feared side effects
  Patients and their carers may often have unfounded fears about medication, such as the idea that antipsychotic drugs are addictive

* Perceived benefit from medication
  Not surprisingly, patients who perceive medication as helpful are more likely to be compliant, even if they experience side effects[188]

IMPROVING COMPLIANCE

* Good relationship between patient and physician

* Providing sufficient information about treatment and potential side effects

* Being sympathetic about patients' complaints regarding side effects and treating side effects vigorously

* Close monitoring of patients' compliance and frequent prompting in a tactful and non-confrontational manner.

* Changing patients from oral to depot medication is a simple and cost-effective approach to covert non-compliance

* Patients are more likely to comply with medication when it is part of a wider package of treatment that offers social and psychological support

* Involving relatives and carers in the treatment plan

* Exploring, and if necessary attempting to modify, patients' and carers' beliefs about illness and medication

* Offering incentives for compliance. Incentives may take different forms, such as establishing patients' clubs at out-patient clinics

Psychosocial interventions

8

Pharmacological treatment on its own has only a moderate impact on the social function of patients with schizophrenia. It must be combined with a broad approach to the many psychological and social problems that afflict schizophrenic patients. The main approaches are outlined below.

Cognitive remediation

Schizophrenic patients manifest a range of neuropsychological abnormalities already discussed in Chapter 5. The goal of the remedial approach is to improve social functioning, and to some extent clinical symptoms, by attempting to ameliorate cognitive deficits.[190] Different treatment programmes have been developed within this framework.[190–192] Initially, specific cognitive defects are identified by tests and observation of the patient's behaviour. The patient is then given different exercises of increasing complexity, which address his or her individual impairment. The results reported so far from clinical trials show improvement in cognitive test performance and social functioning.[190–192]

Cognitive behavioural therapy

The application of cognitive behavioural therapy (CBT) in the treatment of schizophrenic symptoms is based on two assumptions:

- *That schizophrenia emerges in people who, in addition to their biological vulnerability, tend to employ dysfunctional cognitive models of self and environment*

- *That these models are amenable to therapeutic interventions using principles of human learning*

CBT has been used mainly in the treatment of delusions and hallucinations.[193,194] The fundamental elements of this approach can be outlined as:

- *Identification and operational measurement of the target symptoms and behaviours,*

- *Examination of their antecedents and consequences*

- *Formulation, together with the patient, of alternative, more adaptive, explanatory models for the target symptoms*

- *Evaluation of the changes to target symptoms and behaviour*

Evidence accumulating from randomized controlled studies suggests that CBT is effective in reducing positive symptoms overall as well as the frequency of hallucinations and the distress associated with delusions in patients with schizophrenia.[195,196] This effect is not mediated through increased contact with a therapist since patients receiving supportive counselling, as opposed to CBT, do not show comparable improvements.[196] In addition, it appears that the improvement seen in patients during active treatment may be maintained for at least 9–10 months after completion of treatment.[195] In terms of cost effectiveness, CBT appears to reduced the need for hospitalization.[195,196]

Family interventions

It has long been recognized that the emotional relationship of relatives and carers towards patients has a significant impact on the course of schizophrenia. Hostility, critical comments or overinvolvement of relatives and carers (often termed 'high expressed emotion', see pages 20–21) are predictive of higher relapse and rehospitalization rates in patients, whereas warmth and positive remarks seem to have a protective role.[197] At the same time, schizophrenia has a significant impact on the unaffected family members and carers, who often report high levels of distress, social isolation, fears about their personal safety and financial difficulties.[197]

In response to these problems, several family intervention models have been developed:

- *Psychodynamic family therapy*[198]
- *Behavioural family therapy*[198]
- *Relatives' groups*[198]
- *Multiple family groups*[198]

In spite of differences in the techniques used, family interventions programmes have similar components and goals (Table 10).

Some studies have claimed that the combined effect of medication and family intervention can reduce relapse rates by up to 50% compared to medication-only treatment, but there are many studies reporting little or no effect.[199–201] Although there is little evidence that family interventions aid social recovery in schizophrenics, they may reduce the burden on relatives.[202,203] There are few studies comparing the efficacy of different family interventions. Existing data indicate high attrition rates in studies employing psychodynamic family therapy and relatives-

Table 10
Components and goals of family intervention programmes.

Component	Aim
Education about schizophrenia	Increased understanding of the disorder, separating personality from symptoms, acceptance of the possibility of future relapses
Education about treatment	Increased understanding of the role of medication in symptom control and prophylaxis of relapse Improvement of compliance
Communication training and facilitation	Improvement in communication within the family and reduction in friction, critical comments and hostility towards the patient Increase in positive remarks, encouraging respect for individual boundaries within the family
Problem-solving training	Improvement in management of daily living problems and of discrete life events

only groups. The efficacy of multiple family groups seems to be similar to that of individual family groups,[204] making the former a more cost-effective choice.

Psychoeducation

Psychoeducational interventions aim at providing information about the nature and treatment of schizophrenia. They include sessions for patients only, sessions with patients and carers together and carer-only groups.[205] The choice of format depends on the resources available and the social circumstances of the patient. Psychoeducation appears to enhance understanding of the disorder, but information retention is short-lived and the overall impact on patients' and carers' attitudes is limited.[205,206] There is little evidence that psychoeducation produces measurable changes in insight, compliance, rates of relapse or psychosocial functioning.[206] Provision of information to patients and carers is a vital component of good clinical practice but continuous support is also necessary.

Social skills training

Social skills training is the most widely used psychosocial intervention in clinical practice. It grew out of the realization that social deficits may persist even during symptomatic remission. These programmes aim at helping patients to improve their interpersonal behaviour, self-care and adjustment to living in the community. A wide range of techniques is used, including videotapes, psychoeducational material and behavioural modification methods such as positive reinforcement, modelling and role play. Skills acquired during sessions seem to be maintained for long periods,[207] but generalization to natural social settings outside the treatment groups does not occur readily.

Special management problems

9

Pregnancy and the puerperium in schizophrenic patients

Kendell *et al.* (1987)[208] examined the psychiatric effects of childbirth in all women living in the city of Edinburgh during a period of 12 years. Women with a history of affective disorder had a much higher risk of psychiatric admission in the puerperium than those with a history of schizophrenia; in fact, the risk in schizophrenic women was similar to that in women with neurotic illness. Furthermore, there was no significant difference in admission rates among psychotic women during pregnancy than during the previous 15 months. Studies from psychiatric units where mothers and babies are admitted together[209] have also shown that schizophrenic mothers are less likely to require acute admission than mothers with affective disorders.

Nevertheless, the management of schizophrenia during pregnancy presents many problems. For example, Spielvogel and Wile (1992) noted that schizophrenic women with delusions about their pregnancy have a higher risk of obstetric complications than non-delusional women because of their non-compliance with prenatal and perinatal care.[210] The effect of medication on the fetus is another important consideration. Ideally, the patient should remain medication-free during at least the first two trimesters, but this has to be weighed against the risk of deterioration in her mental state. All drugs are potential teratogens, but the risk appears to be more significant with benzodiazepines and lithium than with traditional antipsychotic agents;[211] little information is available yet on the newer antipsychotics.

Studies of high-risk patients show that those children of schizophrenic mothers who had complications during pregnancy and birth have a higher risk themselves of developing the disease than their counterparts whose mothers had an uneventful pregnancy and delivery.[212] The possibility of preventing a further increase in vulnerability in these 'high-risk' children puts a particular premium on the optimum care of pregnant schizophrenic women.

Schizophrenia and depression

At any one time about 25% of schizophrenic patients have depressive symptoms.[213,214] Hafner *et al.* (1999) reported that 81% of schizophrenic patients have depressive symptoms during their first episode and that these symptoms often precede the onset of overt psychosis.[215] Similarly, depressive features are often present in the early phases of subsequent psychotic episodes, during acute episodes and after recovery from psychosis (postpsychotic depression).[216,217] As in affective disorders, the presence of depression in schizophrenia is associated with suicidal ideation and attempted or completed suicide.[218,219]

Depression in schizophrenia needs to be differentiated from:

- **Neuroleptic-induced dysphoria**
  Some patients experience feelings of dysphoria while on neuroleptic agents; this is associated with the presence of extrapyramidal side effects, especially akathisia

- **Neuroleptic-induced akinesia**
  Neuroleptic agents produce a general reduction in psychomotor activity, and patients may complain of tiredness or lack of energy

- **Negative symptoms**
  The negative symptoms of schizophrenia include anhedonia, lack of motivation, loss of interest and anergia. Similar symptoms are also present in depression. However, although in depression there is also persistent low mood, in schizophrenia negative symptoms are associated with blunted affect.[217]

Depressive symptoms during acute episodes improve together with psychotic symptoms, independently of the antipsychotic agent used.[220] There is little to suggest that any particular conventional antipsychotic agent is better than any other for depressive symptoms in schizophrenia.[220–233] There is, however, some evidence that atypical antipsychotic agents may prove more effective.[220] Analysis of pooled data from two double-blind studies comparing risperidone, haloperidol and placebo showed risperidone to be superior in reducing anxiety–depression in patients with chronic schizophrenia.[224] A similar advantage over haloperidol in improving anxiety–depression scores has also been reported in double blind studies of olanzapine and amisulpride.[225,226] Ziprasidone is also superior to placebo in improving depressive symptoms in acute exacerbations of schizophrenia.[227] Clozapine may be particularly effective in reducing suicidality in schizophrenia. Meltzer and Okayli (1995) collected prospective data over a period of 3.5 years in 237 treatment-responsive patients and 183 treatment-resistant patients with schizophrenia and schizoaffective disorder.[228] Suicidality was rated dimensionally from suicidal thoughts to suicidal plans, acts of self-harm and suicide attempts. Suicidality did not differ between the treatment-resistant patients and the treatment-responsive patients. Clozapine appeared to reduce suicidal thoughts but more importantly, it was associated with an 86.4% decrease in all suicide attempts and a significant reduction in the suicide rate.

Antidepressants on their own do not appear to be more effective than placebo in treating depressive symptoms in schizophrenia.[229] However, they may have a role as an adjunct to antipsychotic treatment.[230] Finally, there is limited support regarding the use of mood stabilizers (either lithium or antiepileptic agents) in the treatment of depressive symptoms in schizophrenia.[223,231]

Schizophrenia and violence

Research on the relationship between schizophrenia and violence has focused mainly on criminal behaviour because this is more reliably recorded. Most studies have examined either the prevalence of schizophrenia in a population of offenders or the nature and type of offending in psychiatric populations. Both approaches are fraught with methodological problems, but the picture that emerges suggests that:

- *About 8% of offenders who have either committed or attempted homicide have a diagnosis of schizophrenia[232]*

- *Schizophrenic patients are four times more likely to be involved in violent incidents than people without psychiatric diagnoses[233]*

- *Criminal offending among women, including violent behaviour, seems much higher in schizophrenic patients compared to the general population, in whom the base rate is low, and to non-schizophrenic psychiatric patients[234]*

- **The majority of schizophrenic offenders were known to the psychiatric services but were not receiving treatment at the time of the offence[235]**

- **The peak period of risk for violent acts is 5–10 years after onset[236]**

Criminal acts committed by schizophrenic patients are related to the following features of their illness:

- **Delusions**
  Delusions appear be the most important determinants of violent behaviour, especially those that are intensely held, those for which patients claim to have, or have sought evidence, and those that provoke strong negative affective responses (such as fear or distress). Delusions of control or of religious or paranormal content are more closely related to violence than persecutory delusions[235,237]

- **Hallucinations**
  Hallucinations on their own appear to have little effect on violent behaviour but they may contribute to it in the presence of delusions.[237]

- **Indifference towards the victim**
  Compared to non-psychotic violent offenders, schizophrenic patients are less likely to know or to have been provoked by their victims or express any feelings for them[235]

- **Comorbidity**
  Substance abuse has been repeatedly found to substantially increase the risk of violent behaviour among schizophrenic patients. Rasanen et al. (1998) examined prospective data on criminality and psychiatric disorders over 26 years in an unselected birth cohort.[233] They reported that schizophrenic patients without a history of alcohol abuse were nearly four times more likely than healthy subjects to commit violent crimes. However, for schizophrenic men with comorbid alcoholism, the risk was 25 times higher for violent crimes and nearly 10 times higher for all offending. A similar pattern of increased risk of violence and offending in general has also been found for schizophrenic patients who use illicit drugs[238]

In schizophrenic patients, as in non-psychotic populations, there is an association between antisocial personality traits or disorder and violence. Nolan et al. (1999) found that schizophrenic patients with high rates of psychopathy were more likely to be violent and to have committed more violent and non-violent offenses.[239]

However, it is important to bear in mind that violent and criminal behaviour that could be directly attributable to schizophrenia accounts for only a small proportion of such behaviour within society[240] and that the risk of a schizophrenic patient committing homicide is over 100 less that his or her risk of committing suicide.[232]

Assessment of dangerousness[241]

The accurate prediction of future violence is extremely difficult. Usually, an assessment of dangerousness is requested in patients who have already committed a violent act, and so far the best predictor of future violence has been found to be past violent behaviour. Three major factors need to be taken into account:

THE PATIENT
Important considerations include:[238]

• *the relationship between schizophrenic symptomatology and previous violence;*

• *the degree of clinical response to treatment;*

• *the presence of complicating factors such as abnormal premorbid personality and substance abuse;*

• *the degree of insight shown by the patient;*

• *the patient's views on previous acts of violence; and*

• *the patient's compliance with treatment*

THE ENVIRONMENT
The following aspects should be considered:[242]

• *the degree to which situational factors have influenced previous violent behaviour;*

• *the degree to which predisposing environmental factors have changed since the original violent act; and*

• *the quality of psychiatric aftercare available*

This is particularly important since patients who are well engaged with psychiatric services and are frequent attenders at mental health centres have been shown to be less likely to threaten or commit an act of violence.

POTENTIAL VICTIMS

Important factors include:

- the relationship of the patient to previous victims;

- the possibility of identifying potential victims in advance;

- the quality of the relationship between potential victims and the patient;

- the awareness and views of potential victims of the patient's mental illness and violent behaviour;

- the availability of support for potential victims if they live with the patient, and their easy accessibility to help should they have any concerns.

Estroff et al. (1998) found that people at elevated risk of becoming targets of violence were those in the immediate family of a patient who had frequent contact with the patient and on whom the patient relied financially; mothers who live with their adult schizophrenic children had the highest risk of becoming victims of violence.

Management of a violent patient

Violence as an acute psychiatric emergency[159]

- *Imminent violence*
  It is important to talk calmly to the patient, help him or her recognize the threatening behaviour and set limits in a firm but not confrontational way. Sedative medication is helpful and should be offered. Chlorpromazine and thioridazine are the most sedative of the antipsychotic agents that are commonly used. They can given orally often together with benzodiazepines such as diazepam. Antipsychotic medication, such as zuclopenthixol acetate, can also be administered as an intramuscular injection, ideally with the patient's agreement.

- *Actual violence*
  In situations of actual violence, the objective is to control the violent behaviour by sedation and to ensure the safety of the patient and the staff. At this stage verbal intervention is not helpful and physical restraint becomes necessary. Droperidol can be given intramuscularly or intravenously (5–15 mg every 4–6 hours if necessary). Intravenous benzodiazepines should be used with care because of the danger of respiratory depression. The use of diazepam emulsion (Diazemuls) minimizes the risk of venous thrombophlebitis. Up to 10–20 mg can be given at a rate of 0.5 mg every 30 seconds.[243] After restraint, the patient should be examined and the blood pressure and respiratory rate should be monitored regularly by nursing staff for at least 12 hours. After major or persistent episodes of violence, the plan of management for the patient should be reviewed to obviate further episodes.

Long-term treatment

The treatment of violent patients with schizophrenia is not different from that for any other schizophrenic patient. However, their care should be carefully managed with frequent monitoring of mental state and compliance, and contingency plans should be made in case any deterioration or defaulting with treatment occurs. Some of the atypical antipsychotic agents may be helpful in controlling aggression and may even reduce substance abuse. Clozapine has been shown to have such effects, which may be relatively specific since it is not fully attributable to sedation or overall improvement of psychopathology.[244]

The cost of schizophrenia

10

Schizophrenia is an expensive disorder because:

- *it typically begins early in life at the time of the patient's peak productivity*

- *in many cases, it runs a chronic course that restricts the patient's lifestyle and ability to work*

- *mortality is not particularly high*

- *treatment is only partially effective and is costly*

- *the financial impact of schizophrenia on family members and carers is substantial*

- *both schizophrenic patients and their families experience disadvantages because of the social stigma associated with the disease*

The cost of any disease is a multidimensional concept that can only partly be measured in financial terms. Economists define costs as:

Direct costs	Money spent on providing services to those who are ill
	Expenses incurred by the family members and carers of patients
Indirect costs	Loss of resources that could have been invested in other areas
	Loss of productivity by patients and carers
Intangible costs	Pain and suffering by patients and carers reflected in reduced
	quality of life (not measurable in financial terms)

Direct costs

Prevalence-based studies

Most economic studies measuring the direct cost of schizophrenia are prevalence-based. They are designed to measure costs associated with schizophrenia in a particular country over the period of 1 year. In most developed countries, hospitalization and residential care are the two major contributors; these are followed by day care (Figure 6).

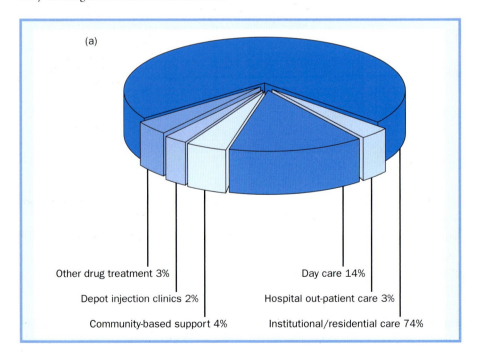

(a)

Other drug treatment 3%

Depot injection clinics 2%

Community-based support 4%

Day care 14%

Hospital out-patient care 3%

Institutional/residential care 74%

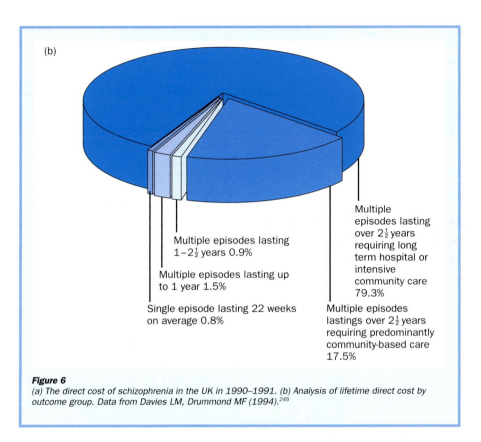

(b)

Multiple episodes lasting 1–2$\frac{1}{2}$ years 0.9%

Multiple episodes lasting up to 1 year 1.5%

Single episode lasting 22 weeks on average 0.8%

Multiple episodes lasting over 2$\frac{1}{2}$ years requiring long term hospital or intensive community care 79.3%

Multiple episodes lastings over 2$\frac{1}{2}$ years requiring predominantly community-based care 17.5%

Figure 6
(a) The direct cost of schizophrenia in the UK in 1990–1991. (b) Analysis of lifetime direct cost by outcome group. Data from Davies LM, Drummond MF (1994).[245]

Drug costs so far have been relatively small, accounting for between 1 and 5% of the direct cost of schizophrenia.[245–247] The new atypical antipsychotic agents are significantly more costly than conventional neuroleptic agents. In the UK, the approximate average monthly cost of treatment with clozapine and risperidone is £168 and £112 respectively, whereas it is less than £30 for haloperidol.[248]

Because of the possibility of inflation of direct costs for treating schizophrenia, there is increased emphasis not just on the clinical evaluation but also on the economic evaluation of new antipsychotic drugs.[249]

There is ongoing debate with regard to the methodology of such cost-effectiveness studies driven either by diverging views among health economists or by diverging policies and priorities among governments or other health management agencies.[249] Expert reviews of existing economic studies of medical interventions have consistently highlighted methodological deficiencies in the majority of such studies.[250,251] These deficiencies include lack of prospective data collected as part of randomized, controlled clinical trials and the over-reliance on 'before and after' designs, small and highly selected patient samples and short periods of data collection. Furthermore, since a significant proportion of cost-effectiveness studies are sponsored by the pharmaceutical industry, the potential for bias cannot be ignored.

Within this framework, clozapine and risperidone are the two atypical antipsychotic agents whose cost-effectiveness has been most extensively examined. It would appear that clozapine would be cost saving or at least cost neutral in the treatment of drug resistant schizophrenia in spite its higher acquisition cost.[248] Clozapine appears to reduce in-patient care costs with marked improvement in scores on scales of psychopathology and social disability.[252] A similar pattern has been reported for risperidone in the treatment of chronic schizophrenia, for which the existing evidence suggests that it may cost neutral or may even reduce hospitalization and thus overall costs.[253,254] Initial data on olanzapine suggest that it is probably cost neutral but,

like clozapine and risperidone, it may produce better clinical outcomes than typical antipsychotics.[254]

Incidence-based studies

Average costs of treatment for schizophrenia do not address the issue of variability in severity and outcome of the disorder. Incidence-based studies assess the future (lifetime) cost of treating all new cases of schizophrenia arising during a given period of time (usually 1 year) and allow the calculation of the distribution of costs according to severity of illness. Although patients with chronic schizophrenia represent less than half of a 1-year incidence cohort, their care absorbs 97% of the total lifetime direct costs.[245]

The overall direct costs of schizophrenia are comparable to those of other psychiatric disorders such as depression. According to a UK study, the direct costs of depression were estimated at £417 million, compared to £310 million for schizophrenia.[255] However, since the prevalence of depression is at least four times that of schizophrenia,[256] the average cost per patient is much higher for schizophrenia.

Direct and indirect family costs

The majority of schizophrenic patients do not require long-term institutionalized care and so live at home, often with their family.

Establishing the cost of schizophrenia for the families is very important especially in the present climate that favours community care for the mentally ill; indeed, to some extent the move to community care represents a shift of the burden of care from collectively funded agencies to the family. This family burden can be both financial (in terms of money and time contributed by carers) and emotional.

The accurate estimation of the cost to families is very difficult. One study in the USA found that most of the carers were ageing parents who devoted, on average, 15 hours per week and spent about $US3540 per year in the care of their schizophrenic family member.[257] This estimate was independent of the family's financial ability to afford the patient's care. A UK survey reported that the expense of caring for a schizophrenic member led one in 10 families to financial difficulties.[245] A significant proportion of family members either had to take time off or even had to stop work to look after the affected member.[245]

Indirect costs

The indirect costs of schizophrenia reflect the loss in productivity of patients and carers that result from illness and the loss of resources that could have been invested elsewhere.

Measuring these indirect costs is a complex task because:

- *Accurate information on the loss of productivity of carers is not readily available*

- *Schizophrenic patients represent a heterogeneous group, and the loss of potential productivity varies widely according to their sex, age at onset, cultural background and education*

- *Disease-independent factors, such as the general level of unemployment, affect potential productivity and have to be taken into account*

- *It is difficult to assign monetary value to various forms of work, such as domestic activities*

- *Potential gains to society from the investment in other areas of resources currently allocated to schizophrenia can only be guessed at*

Nevertheless, the assessment of earnings lost as a result of the inability of schizophrenic patients to work because of their illness provides some indication of the magnitude of indirect costs. In a UK study, the annual indirect costs incurred through productivity loss by patients were thought to exceed £1.7 billion, which is at least four times higher than the direct costs estimated in the same study.[245]

Useful addresses in the UK

Institute of Psychiatry
De Crespigny Park
Denmark Hill
London SE5 8AF
Tel: 020 7703 5411
(General enquiries)
Tel: 020 7919 3536
Fax: 020 7701 9044

National Psychosis Unit
Maudsley Hospital
Denmark Hill
London SE5 PAZ
Tel: 020 7703 6091

Afro-Caribbean Mental Health Association
35–37 Electric Avenue
London SW9 8JP
Tel: 020 7737 3603

Making Space
(Yorkshire and NW England)
46 Allen Street, Warrington
Cheshire WA2 7JB
Tel: 01925 571680

MIND
National Association for Mental Health
Granta House
15/19 Broadway, Stratford
London E15 4BQ
Tel: 020 8522 1728
Fax: 020 8522 1725

The National Council of Voluntary
Organizations (NCVO)
Regents' Wharf
8 All Saints Street
London N7 9RL
Tel: 020 7713 6161

National Schizophrenia Fellowship
NSF National Office
28 Castle Street
Kingston-upon-Thames
Surrey KT1 1SS
Tel: 020 8547 3937
Fax: 020 8547 3862
Advice Line: 020 8974 6814

Richmond Fellowship for Community
Mental Health
8 Addison Road
Kensington
London W14 8DL
Tel: 020 7603 6373

Royal College of Psychiatrists
17 Belgrave Square
London SW1X 8PG
Tel: 020 7325 2351

The Samaritans
10 The Grove
Slough
Berks SL1 1QP
Tel: 01753 531001

SANE (Schizophrenia – A National
Emergency)
199–205 Old Marylebone Road
London NW1 5QP
Tel: 020 7724 8000
SANELINE: 020 7724 8000

Appendix
Diagnostic criteria and clinical subtypes of schizophrenia

ICD-10

At least one of the symptoms (a)–(d) or at least two of the symptoms (e)–(i) should have been present during a period of a month or more:

(a) thought echo, thought insertion or withdrawal, and thought broadcasting

(b) delusions of control, influence, or passivity, clearly referred to body or limb movements or specific thoughts, actions or sensations; delusional perception

(c) hallucinatory voices giving a running commentary on the patient's behaviour, or discussing the patient among themselves, or other types of hallucinatory voices coming from some part of the body

(d) persistent delusions of other kinds that are culturally inappropriate and completely impossible, such as religious or political identity, or superhuman powers and abilities

(e) persistent hallucinations in any modality, accompanied either by fleeting or half-formed delusions without clear affective component, or by persistent overvalued ideas, or occurring every day for weeks or months on end

(f) breaks or interpolations in the train of thought, resulting in incoherence or irrelevant speech, or neologisms

(g) catatonic behaviour, such as excitement, posturing, or waxy flexibility, negativism, mutism and stupor

(h) 'negative' symptoms such as marked apathy, paucity of speech and blunting or incongruity of emotional responses, usually resulting in social withdrawal and lowering of social performance; it must be clear that they are not due to depression or to neuroleptic medication

(i) a significant and consistent change in the overall quality of some aspects of personal behaviour, manifest as loss of interest, aimlessness, idleness, a self-absorbed attitude and social withdrawal.

Clinical subtypes of schizophrenia
DSM IV

Type	Diagnostic criteria
Paranoid	Preoccupation with one or more delusions or frequent auditory hallucinations
	None of the following should be prominent: disorganized speech, disorganized or catatonic behaviour, or flat or inappropriate affect
Disorganized	Prominent disorganized speech and behaviour, flat or inappropriate affect
	Should not meet any criteria for the catatonic type
Catatonic	At least two of the following: motor immobility as evidenced by cataplexy or stupor; excessive motor activity apparently purposeless and not influenced by external stimuli; peculiarities of voluntary movement as evidenced by posturing, stereotyped movements, prominent mannerisms or prominent grimacing; echolalia or echopraxia
Undifferentiated	Does not meet the criteria for the above types
Residual	Absence of prominent delusions, hallucinations, disorganized speech and grossly disorganized or catatonic behaviour; continuing evidence of the disturbance indicated by the presence of negative symptoms or two or more of the above symptoms in an attenuated form

DSM IV

A. *Characteristic symptoms: At least two of the following symptoms, each present for a significant portion of the time during a one month period:*
   (a) delusions
   (b) hallucinations
   (c) disorganized or catatonic behaviour
   (d) grossly disorganized or catatonic behaviour
   (e) negative symptoms, i.e. affective flattening, allege or avocation.

B. *Social/occupational dysfunction: For a significant portion of the time since the onset of the disturbance, one or more major areas of functioning such as work, interpersonal relationships or self care are markedly below the level achieved prior to the onset.*

C. *Duration. Continuous signs of the disturbance persist for at least 6 months. This 6-month period must include at least 1 month of symptoms that meet criterion A and may include periods of prodromal and residual symptoms. During these prodromal or residual periods the signs of the disturbance may be manifested by only negative symptoms or two or more symptoms listed in criterion A present in attenuated form.*

D. *Schizoaffective and mood disorder exclusion: Schizoaffective and mood disorders have been ruled out because either (1) no major depressive, manic or mixed episodes have occurred concurrently with the active-phase symptoms; or (2) if mood episodes have occurred during active-phase symptoms, their total duration has been brief relative to the duration of the active and residual periods.*

E. *Substance/general medical condition exclusion: The disturbance is not due to the direct physiological effects of a substance (e.g. drug of abuse, a medication) or a general medical condition.*

F. *Relationship to a pervasive developmental disorder: If there is a history of autistic disorder or another pervasive developmental disorder, the additional diagnosis of schizophrenia is made only if prominent delusions or hallucinations are also present for at least one month.*

ICD-10

Type	Diagnostic criteria
Paranoid	Delusions, usually accompanied by hallucinations, predominate. Disturbances of affect, volition and speech, and catatonic symptoms are not prominent
Hebephrenia	Mood is inappropriate and speech disorganized and incoherent; negative symptoms develop rapidly; delusions and hallucinations may be present but usually not prominent; can be used in adolescents or young adults
Catatonic	Prominent psychomotor disturbances or either catatonic excitement, stupor or posturing
Undifferentiated	Does not conform with above subtypes and no particular set of symptoms predominates

These subtypes are based on clinical presentation and do not reliably predict either treatment response or prognosis. Nevertheless, many psychiatrists find them useful as a descriptive shorthand. The catatonic subtype has become steadily less common in industrial countries since the beginning of the century while the paranoid subtype has become more common; the reasons for this change are unknown.

References

World Health Organization. *ICD-10 Classification of Mental and Behavioural Disorders. Clinical Conditions and Diagnostic Guidelines.* Geneva: WHO, 1992.
American Psychiatric Association. *Diagnostic and Statistical Manual of Mental Disorders*, 4th edn. Washington DC: American Psychiatric Association, 1994.

References

1. McEvoy JP, Freter S, Everett G *et al.* Insight and the clinical outcome of schizophrenic patients. *J Nerv Ment Dis* 1989; **177**: 48–51.

2. Liddle PF. The symptoms of chronic schizophrenia. A re-examination of the positive–negative dichotomy. *Br J Psychiatry* 1987; **151**: 145–151.

3. Jones P, Rodgers B, Murray R, Marmot M. Child development risk factors for adult schizophrenia in the British 1946 birth cohort. *Lancet* 1994; **344**: 1398–1402.

4. Jones P, Murray R, Rodgers B. Childhood risk factors for adult schizophrenia in a general population birth cohort at 43 years. In: Mednick SA, Hollister JM, eds. *Neurol Development and Schizophrenia.* New York: Plenum Press, 1995.

5. Hafner H, Nowotny B. Epidemiology of early-onset schizophrenia. *Eur Arch Psychiatry Clin Neurosci* 1995; **245**: 80–92.

6. World Health Organization. *Report of the International Pilot Study of Schizophrenia.* Geneva, 1973.

7. Bleuler M. The long-term course of schizophrenic psychoses. *Psychol Med* 1974; **4**: 244–254.

8. Ram R, Bromet EJ, Eaton WW *et al.* The natural course of schizophrenia: a review of first-admission studies. *Schizophr Bull* 1992; **18**: 185–207.

9. Shepherd M, Watt D, Falloon I, Smeeton N. The natural history of schizophrenia: a five-year follow-up study of outcome and prediction in a representative sample of schizophrenics. *Psychol Med Monogr Suppl* 1989; **15**: 1–46.

10. Ciompi L. Catamnestic long-term study of the course of life and aging in schizophrenics. *Schizophr Bull* 1980; **6**: 606–618.

11. Sartorius N, Jablensky A, Korten A *et al.* Early manifestations and first-contact incidence of schizophrenia in different cultures. A preliminary report on the initial evaluation phase of the WHO Collaborative Study on determinants of outcome of severe mental disorders. *Psychol Med* 1986; **16**: 909–928.

12. Robinson D, Woerner MG, Alvir JM *et al.* Predictors of relapse following response from a first episode of schizophrenia or schizoaffective disorder. *Arch Gen Psychiatry* 1999; **56**: 241–247.

13. Ohmori T, Ito K, Abekawa T, Koyama T. Psychotic relapse and maintenance therapy in paranoid schizophrenia: a 15 year follow up. *Eur Arch Psychiatry Clin Neurosci* 1999; **249**: 73–78.

14. Tsuang MT, Woolson RF, Fleming JA. Premature deaths in schizophrenia and affective disorders: an analysis of survival curves and variables affecting the shortened survival. *Arch Gen Psychiatry* 1980; **37**: 979–983.

15. Allebeck P. Schizophrenia: a life shortening disease. *Schizophr Bull* 1989; **15**: 81–89.

16. Wiersma D, Nienhuis FJ, Slooff CJ, Giel R. Natural course of schizophrenic disorders: a 15-year followup of a Dutch incidence cohort. *Schizophr Bull* 1998; **24**: 75–85.

17. Heila H, Isometsa ET, Henriksson MM *et al.* Suicide and schizophrenia: a nationwide psychological autopsy study on age- and sex-specific clinical characteristics of 92 suicide victims with schizophrenia. *Am J Psychiatry* 1997; **154**: 1235–1242.

18. Fenton WS, McGlashan TH, Victor BJ, Blyler CR. Symptoms, subtype, and suicidality in patients with schizophrenia spectrum disorders. *Am J Psychiatry* 1997; **154**: 199–204.

19. Tsuang MT, Simpson JC, Kronfold Z. Subtypes of drug abuse with psychosis. *Arch Gen Psychiatry* 1982; **39**: 141–147.

20. Jablensky A, Sartorius N, Ernberg G *et al.* Schizophrenia: manifestations, incidence and course in different cultures. A World Health Organization ten-country study. *Psychol Med Monogr Suppl* 1992; **20**: 1–97.

21. Hare E. Schizophrenia as a recent disease. *Br J Psychiatry* 1988; **153**: 521–531.

22. Der G, Gupta S, Murray RM. Is schizophrenia disappearing? *Lancet* 1990; **335**: 513–516.

23. Hafner H, Maurer K, Loffler W *et al.* The epidemiology of early schizophrenia. Influence of age and gender on onset and early course. *Br J Psychiatry Suppl* 1994; **23**: 29–38.

24. Hagnell O, Ojesjo L, Otterbeck L, Rorsman B. Prevalence of mental disorders, personality traits and mental complaints in the Lundby study. A point prevalence study of the 1957 Lundby cohort of 2,612 inhabitants of a geographically defined area who were re-examined in 1972 regardless of domicile. *Scand J Soc Med Suppl* 1994; **50**: 1–77.

25. Freeman H. Schizophrenia and city residence. *Br J Psychiatry Suppl* 1994; **23**: 39–50.

26. Loffler W, Hafner H. Ecological pattern of first admitted schizophrenics in two German cities over 25 years. *Soc Sci Med* 1999; **49**: 93–108.

27. Aro S, Aro H, Keskimaki I. Socio-economic mobility among patients with schizophrenia or major affective disorder. A 17-year retrospective follow-up. *Br J Psychiatry* 1995; **166**: 759–767.

28. McNaught AS, Jeffreys SE, Harvey CA *et al.* The Hampstead Schizophrenia Survey 1991. II: Incidence and migration in inner London. *Br J Psychiatry* 1997; **170**: 307–311.

29. Torrey EF, Bowler AE, Clark K. Urban birth and residence as risk factors for psychoses: an analysis of 1880 data. *Schizophr Res* 1997; **25**: 169–176.

30. Mortensen PB, Pedersen CB, Westergaard T *et al.* Effects of family history and place and season of birth on the risk of

schizophrenia. *N Engl J Med* 1999; **340**: 603–608.

31. Harrison G, Glazebrook C, Brewin J *et al.* Increased incidence of psychotic disorders in migrants from the Caribbean to the United Kingdom. *Psychol Med* 1997; **27**: 799–806.

32. Haasen C, Lambert M, Mass R, Krausz M. Impact of ethnicity on the prevalence of psychiatric disorders among migrants in Germany. *Ethnic Health* 1998; **3**: 159–165.

33. Bhugra D, Leff J, Mallett R *et al.* Incidence and outcome of schizophrenia in whites, African–Caribbeans and Asians in London. *Psychol Med* 1997; **27**: 791–798.

34. Burnett R, Mallett R, Bhugra D *et al.* The first contact of patients with schizophrenia with psychiatric services: social factors and pathways to care in a multi-ethnic population. *Psychol Med* 1999; **29**: 475–483.

35. Odegaard O. Fertility of psychiatric first admissions in Norway, 1936–75. *Acta Psychiatr Scand* 1980; **62**: 212–220.

36. Murray RM, McGuffin P. Genetic aspects of psychiatric disorders. In: Kendell RE, Zealley AK, eds. *Companion to Psychiatric Studies* 5th edn. Edinburgh: Churchill-Livingstone, 1993, 227–261.

37. Kendler KS, McGuire M, Gruenberg AM, Walsh D. Clinical heterogeneity in schizophrenia and the pattern of psychopathology in relatives: results from an epidemiologically based family study. *Acta Psychiatr Scand* 1994; **89**: 294–300.

38. Sham PC, Jones P, Russell A *et al.* Age at onset, sex, and familial psychiatric morbidity in schizophrenia. Camberwell Collaborative Psychosis Study. *Br J Psychiatry* 1994; **165**: 466–473.

39. Cannon TD, Kaprio J, Lonnqvist J *et al.* The genetic epidemiology of schizophrenia in a Finnish twin cohort. A population-based modelling study. *Arch Gen Psychiatry* 1998; **55**: 67–74.

40. Neuropsychiatric genetics. (Entire issue). *Am J Med Genet* 1999; **88**: 215–278.

41. McNeil TF. Perinatal risk factors and schizophrenia: selective review and methodological concerns. *Epidemiol Rev* 1995; **17**: 107–112.

42. McGrath J, Murray R. Risk factors for schizophrenia: from Conception to Birth. In: Hirsch SR, Weinberger DR, eds. *Schizophrenia*. Oxford: Blackwell Science, 1995, 187–205.

43. Cannon TD, Mednick SA, Parnas J *et al*. Developmental brain abnormalities in the offspring of schizophrenic mothers. I. Contributions of genetic and perinatal factors. *Arch Gen Psychiatry* 1993; **50**: 551–564.

44. Stefanis N, Frangou S, Yakeley J *et al*. Hippocampal volume reduction in schizophrenia: Effects of genetic risk and pregnancy and birth complications. *Biol Psychiatry* 1999; **46**: 697–702.

45. Jones P, Murray RM. The genetics of schizophrenia is the genetics of neurodevelopment. *Br J Psychiatry* 1991; **158**: 615–623.

46. Brown GW. Experiences of discharged chronic schizophrenic mental hospital patients in various types of living group. *Millbank Memorial Fund Q* 1959; **37**: 105–131.

47. Bebbington P, Kuipers L. The clinical utility of expressed emotion in schizophrenia. *Acta Psychiatr Scand Suppl* 1994; **382**: 46–53.

48. Bebbington P, Kuipers L. The predictive utility of expressed emotion in schizophrenia: an aggregate analysis. *Psychol Med* 1994; **24**: 707–718.

49. Vaughn C, Leff J. The measurement of expressed emotion in the families of psychiatric patients. *Br J Soc Clin Psychol* 1976; **2**: 157–165.

50. Norman RM, Malla AK. Stressful life events and schizophrenia. I: A review of the research. *Br J Psychiatry* 1993; **162**: 161–166.

51. Norman RM, Malla AK. Stressful life events and schizophrenia. II: Conceptual and methodological issues. *Br J Psychiatry* 1993; **162**: 166–174.

52. Jacobs S, Myers J. Recent life events and acute schizophrenic psychosis: A controlled study. *J Nerv Ment Dis* 1976; **162**: 75–87.

53. Bebbington P, Wilkins S, Jones P *et al*. Life events and psychosis. Initial results from the Camberwell Collaborative Psychosis Study. *Br J Psychiatry* 1993; **162**: 72–79.

54. Addington J, Addington D. Effect of substance misuse in early psychosis. *Br J Psychiatry Suppl* 1998; **172**: 134–136.

55. Allebeck P, Adamsson C, Engstrom A, Rydberg U. Cannabis and schizophrenia: a longitudinal study of cases treated in Stockholm County. *Acta Psychiatr Scand* 1993; **88**: 21–24.

56. Andreasson S, Allebeck P, Engstrom A, Rydberg U. Cannabis and schizophrenia. A longitudinal study of Swedish conscripts. *Lancet* 1987; **ii**: 1483–1486.

57. Andreasson S, Allebeck P, Rydberg U. Schizophrenia in users and nonusers of cannabis. A longitudinal study in Stockholm County. *Acta Psychiatr Scand* 1989; **79**: 505–510.

58. Lawrie SM, Abukmeil SS. Brain abnormality in schizophrenia. A systematic and quantitative review of volumetric magnetic resonance imaging studies. *Br J Psychiatry* 1998; **172**: 110–120.

59. Vita A, Dieci M, Giobbio GM *et al.* CT scan abnormalities and outcome of chronic schizophrenia. *Am J Psychiatry* 1991; **148**: 1577–1579.

60. Wright IC, Rabe-Hesketh S, Woodruff PWR *et al.* Meta-analysis of regional brain volumes in schizophrenia. *Am J Psychiatry* 1999; in press.

61. Nelson MD, Saykin AJ, Flashman LA, Riordan HJ. Hippocampal volume reduction in schizophrenia as assessed by magnetic resonance imaging. A meta-analytic study. *Arch Gen Psychiatry* 1998; **55**: 433–440.

62. Gur RE, Pearlson G. Neuroimaging in schizophrenia research. *Schizophr Bull* 1993; **19**: 337–353.

63. Chakos MH, Lieberman JA, Alvir J *et al.* Caudate nuclei volumes in schizophrenic patients treated with typical antipsychotics or clozapine. *Lancet* 1995; **345**: 456–457.

64. Vita A, Dieci M, Giobbio GM *et al.* Time course of cerebral ventricular enlargement in schizophrenia supports the hypothesis of its neurodevelopmental nature. *Schizophr Res* 1997; **23**: 25–30.

65. Jaskiw GE, Juliano DM, Goldberg TE *et al.* Cerebral ventricular enlargement in schizophreniform disorder does not progress. A seven year follow-up study. *Schizophr Res* 1994; **14**: 23–28.

66. Gur RE, Cowell P, Turetsky BI *et al.* A follow-up magnetic resonance imaging study of schizophrenia. Relationship of neuroanatomical changes to clinical and neurobehavioral measures. *Arch Gen Psychiatry* 1998; **55**: 145–152.

67. DeLisi LE, Sakuma M, Shuming G, Kushner M. Association of brain structural change with the heterogeneous course of schizophrenia from early childhood through five years subsequent to a first hospitalization. *Psychiatry Res* 1998; **84**: 75–88.

68. Rapoport JL, Giedd J, Kumra S *et al.* Childhood-onset schizophrenia. Progressive ventricular change during adolescence. *Arch Gen Psychiatry* 1997; **54**: 897–903.

69. Rapoport JL, Giedd JN, Blumenthal J *et al.* Progressive cortical change during adolescence in childhood-onset schizophrenia. A longitudinal magnetic resonance imaging study. *Arch Gen Psychiatry* 1999; **56**: 649–654.

70. Harrison PJ. The neuropathology of schizophrenia. A critical review of the data and their interpretation. *Brain* 1999; **122**: 593–624.

71. Liddle PF, Friston KJ, Frith CD *et al.* Patterns of cerebral blood flow in schizophrenia. *Br J Psychiatry* 1992; **160**: 179–186.

72. Shergill S, Brammer MJ, Williams SCR *et al.* Auditory hallucinations: Mapping the neural networks involved using fMRI. *Arch Gen Psychiatry* 1999; in press.

73. Ffytche DH, Howard RJ, Brammer MJ *et al.* The anatomy of conscious vision: an fMRI study of visual hallucinations. *Nat Neurosci* 1998; **1**: 738–742.

74. Spence SA, Brooks DJ, Hirsch SR *et al.* A PET study of voluntary movement in schizophrenic patients experiencing passivity phenomena (delusions of alien control). *Brain* 1997; **120**: 1997–2011.

75. Velakoulis D, Pantelis C. What have we learned from functional imaging studies in schizophrenia? The role of frontal, striatal and temporal areas. *Aust NZJ Psychiatry* 1996; **30**: 195–209.

76. Bullmore ET, Frangou S, Murray RM. The dysplastic net hypothesis: an integration of developmental and disconnectivity theories of schizophrenia. *Schizophr Res* 1997; **28**: 143–156.

77. Stanley JA, Williamson PC, Drost DJ *et al.* An in vivo proton magnetic resonance spectroscopy study of schizophrenia patients. *Schizophr Bull* 1996; **22**: 597–609.

78. Cecil KM, Lenkinski RE, Gur RE, Gur RC. Proton magnetic resonance spectroscopy in the frontal and temporal lobes of neuroleptic naive patients with schizophrenia. *Neuropsychopharmacology* 1999; **20**: 131–140.

79. Deicken RF, Zhou L, Schuff N *et al.* Hippocampal neuronal dysfunction in schizophrenia as measured by proton magnetic resonance spectroscopy. *Biol Psychiatry* 1998; **43**: 483–488.

80. Deicken RF, Zhou L, Schuff N, Weiner MW. Proton magnetic resonance spectroscopy of the anterior cingulate region in schizophrenia. *Schizophr Res* 1997; **27**: 65–71.

81. Lim KO, Adalsteinsson E, Spielman D *et al.* Proton magnetic resonance spectroscopic imaging of cortical gray and white matter in schizophrenia. *Arch Gen Psychiatry* 1998; **55**: 346–352.

82. Stanley JA, Williamson PC, Drost DJ *et al.* An in vivo proton magnetic resonance spectroscopy study of schizophrenia patients. *Schizophr Bull* 1996; **22**: 597–609.

83. Maier M, Ron MA. Hippocampal age-related changes in schizophrenia: a proton magnetic resonance spectroscopy study. *Schizophr Res* 1996; **22**: 5–17.

84. Buckley PF, Moore C, Long H *et al.* 1H-magnetic resonance spectroscopy of the left temporal and frontal lobes in schizophrenia: clinical, neurodevelopmental, and cognitive correlates. *Biol Psychiatry* 1994; **36**: 792–800.

85. Shioiri T, Hamakawa H, Kato T *et al.* Proton magnetic resonance spectroscopy of the basal ganglia in patients with schizophrenia: a preliminary report. *Schizophr Res* 1996; **22**: 19–26.

86. Choe BY, Kim KT, Suh TS *et al.* 1H magnetic resonance spectroscopy characterization of neuronal dysfunction in drug-naive, chronic schizophrenia. *Acad Radiol* 1994; **1**: 211–216.

87. Stanley JA, Williamson PC, Drost DJ *et al.* An in vivo study of the prefrontal cortex of schizophrenic patients at different stages of illness via phosphorus magnetic resonance spectroscopy. *Arch Gen Psychiatry* 1995; **52**: 399–406.

88. Hinsberger AD, Williamson PC, Carr TJ *et al.* Magnetic resonance imaging volumetric and phosphorus 31 magnetic resonance spectroscopy measurements in schizophrenia. *J Psychiatry Neurosci* 1997; **22**: 111–117.

89. Frangou S, Williams SCR. Magnetic resonance spectroscopy in psychiatry: basic principles and applications. *Br Med Bull* 1996; **52**: 474–485.

90. Keshavan MS, Pettegrew JW, Panchalingam KS *et al.* Phosphorus 31 magnetic resonance spectroscopy detects altered brain metabolism before onset of schizophrenia. *Arch Gen Psychiatry* 1991; **48**: 1112–1113.

91. Sunahara RK, Seeman P, Van Tol HH, Niznik HB. Dopamine receptors and antipsychotic drug response. *Br J Psychiatry Suppl* 1993; **22**: 31–38.

92. Farde L. Brain imaging of schizophrenia: the dopamine hypothesis. *Schizophr Res* 1997; **28**: 157–162.

93. Kerwin R, Owen M. Genetics of novel therapeutic targets in schizophrenia. *Br J Psychiatry* 1999; **174**: 1–4.

94. Meltzer HY. The role of serotonin in schizophrenia and the place of serotonin–dopamine antagonist antipsychotics. *J Clin Psychopharmacol* 1995; **15(suppl)**: 2S–3S.

95. Royston MC, Simpson MDC. Post-mortem neurochemistry of schizophrenia. In: Kerwin R, Dawbarn D, McCulloch J, Tamminga C, eds. *Neurobiology and Psychiatry*. Cambridge: Cambridge University Press, 1991, 1–14.

96. Bleuler E. *Dementia Praecox or the Group of Schizophrenias*. New York: International Universities Press, 1950.

97. Heinrichs RW, Zakzanis KK. Neurocognitive deficit in schizophrenia. A quantitative review of the evidence. *Neuropsychology* 1998; **12**: 426–445.

98. Cannon M, Jones P, Huttunen MO *et al.* School performance in Finnish children and later development of schizophrenia: a population-based longitudinal study. *Arch Gen Psychiatry* 1999; **56**: 457–463.

99. Walker EF, Lewine RR, Neumann C. Childhood behavioral characteristics and adult brain morphology in schizophrenia. *Schizophr Res* 1996; **22**: 93–101.

100. Nopoulos P, Flashman L, Flaum M *et al.* Stability of cognitive functioning early in the course of schizophrenia. *Schizophr Res* 1994; **14**: 29–37.

101. Censits DM, Ragland JD, Gur RC, Gur RE. Neuropsychological evidence supporting a neurodevelopmental model of schizophrenia: a longitudinal study. *Schizophr Res* 1997; **24**: 289–298.

102. DeLisi LE, Tew W, Xie S *et al.* A prospective follow-up study of brain morphology and cognition in first-episode schizophrenic patients: preliminary findings. *Biol Psychiatry* 1995; **38**: 349–360.

103. Robinson DG, Woerner MG, Alvir JM *et al.* Predictors of treatment response from a first episode of schizophrenia or schizoaffective disorder. *Am J Psychiatry* 1999; **156**: 544–549.

104. Robinson D, Woerner MG, Alvir JM *et al.* Predictors of relapse following response from a first episode of schizophrenia or schizoaffective disorder. *Arch Gen Psychiatry* 1999; **56:** 241–247.

105. Green MF. What are the functional consequences of neurocognitive deficits in schizophrenia? *Am J Psychiatry* 1996; **153:** 321–330.

106. Kremen WS, Buka SL, Seidman LJ *et al.* IQ decline during childhood and adult psychotic symptoms in a community sample: a 19-year longitudinal study. *Am J Psychiatry* 1998; **155:** 672–677.

107. Jones P, Rodgers B, Murray R, Marmot M. Child development risk factors for adult schizophrenia in the British 1946 birth cohort. *Lancet* 1994; **344:** 1398–1402.

108. Russell AJ, Munro JC, Jones PB *et al.* Schizophrenia and the myth of intellectual decline. *Am J Psychiatry* 1997; **154:** 635–639.

109. Waddington JL, Youssef HA. Cognitive dysfunction in chronic schizophrenia followed prospectively over 10 years and its longitudinal relationship to the emergence of tardive dyskinesia. *Psychol Med* 1996; **26:** 681–688.

110. Harvey PD, Silverman JM, Mohs RC *et al.* Cognitive decline in late-life schizophrenia: a longitudinal study of geriatric chronically hospitalized patients. *Biol Psychiatry* 1999; **45:** 32–40.

111. Heaton RK, Crowley TJ. Effect of psychiatric disorders and their somatic treatments on neuropsychological test results. In: Filskov S, Boll TJ, eds. *Handbook of Clinical Neuropsychology.* New York: John Wiley and Sons, 1981, 481–525.

112. Mortimer AM. Cognitive function in schizophrenia: do neuroleptics make a difference? *Pharmacol Biochem Behav* 1997; **56:** 789–795.

113. Bilder RM, Turkel E, Lipschutz-Broch L, Lieberman JA. Antipsychotic medication effects on neuropsychological functions. *Psychopharm Bull* 1992; **28:** 353–366.

114. Spohn HE, Strauss ME. Relation of neuroleptic and anticholinergic medication to cognitive functions in schizophrenia. *J Abnorm Psychol* 1989; **98:** 367–380.

115. Sweeney JA, Haas GL, Keilp JG, Long M. Evaluation of the stability of neuropsychological functioning after acute episodes of schizophrenia: one-year followup study. *Psychiatry Res* 1991; **38:** 63–76.

116. Sweeney JA, Keilp JG, Haas GL *et al.*
Relationships between medication
treatments and neuropsychological test
performance in schizophrenia. *Psychiatry
Res* 1991; **37**: 297–308.

117. Classen W, Laux G. Sensorimotor and
cognitive performance of schizophrenic
inpatients treated with haloperidol,
flupenthixol, or clozapine.
Pharmacopsychiatry 1988; **21**: 295–297.

118. Meltzer H, McGurk SR. The effects of
clozapine, risperidone and olanzapine on
cognitive function in schizophrenia.
Schizophr Bull 1999; **25**: 233–255.

119. Sax KW, Strakowski SM, Keck PE Jr.
Attentional improvement following
quetiapine fumarate treatment in
schizophrenia. *Schizophr Res* 1998; **33**:
151–155.

120. Delay J, Deniker O. Characteristiques
psychophysiologiques des médicaments
neuroleptiques. In: Garattini J, Ghetti V,
eds. *The Psychotropic Drugs.* Amsterdam:
Elsevier, 1957, 485–501.

121. Wagstaff AJ, Bryson HM. Clozapine. A
review of its pharmacological properties
and therapeutic use in patients with
schizophrenia who are unresponsive to or
intolerant of classical antipsychotic agents.
CNS Drugs 1994; **4**: 370–400.

122. Barnes TRE, McPhillips MA. Critical
analysis and comparison of the side effect
and safety profile of the new antipsychotics.
Br J Psychiatry 1999; **174**: 34–43.

123. Pickar D. Prospects for pharmacotherapy of
schizophrenia. *Lancet* 1995; **345**: 557–562.

124. Davies A, Adena MA, Keks NA *et al.*
Risperidone versus haloperidol: I. Meta-
analysis of efficacy and safety. *Clin Ther*
1998; **20**: 58–71.

125. Marder SR, Davis JM, Chouinard G. The
effects of risperidone on the five
dimensions of schizophrenia derived by
factor analysis: combined results of the
North American trials. *J Clin Psychiatry*
1997; **58**: 538–546.

126. Chouinard G, Kopala L, Labelle A *et al.*
Phase-IV multicentre clinical study of
risperidone in the treatment of outpatients
with schizophrenia. The RIS-CAN-3 Study
Group. *Can J Psychiatry* 1998; **43**:
1018–1025.

127. Olanzapine, sertindole and schizophrenia.
Drug Ther Bull 1999; **35**: 81–83.

128. Leucht S, Pitschel-Walz G, Abraham D,
Kissling W. Efficacy and extrapyramidal
side-effects of the new antipsychotics
olanzapine, quetiapine, risperidone, and

sertindole compared to conventional antipsychotics and placebo. A meta-analysis of randomized controlled trials. *Schizophr Res* 1999; **35**: 51–68.

129. Peuskens J, Link CG. A comparison of quetiapine and chlorpromazine in the treatment of schizophrenia. *Acta Psychiatr Scand* 1997; **96**: 265–273.

130. Arvanitis LA, Miller BG. Multiple fixed doses of 'Seroquel' (quetiapine) in patients with acute exacerbation of schizophrenia: a comparison with haloperidol and placebo. The Seroquel Trial 13 Study Group. *Biol Psychiatry* 1997; **42**: 233–246.

131. Misra LK, Erpenbach JE, Hamlyn H, Fuller WC. Quetiapine: a new atypical antipsychotic. *SDJ Med* 1998; **51**: 189–193.

132. Scatton B, Claustre Y, Cudennec A *et al.* Amisulpride: from animal pharmacology to therapeutic action. *Int Clin Psychopharmacol* 1997; **12(suppl 2)**: S29–S36.

133. Trichard C, Paillere-Martinot ML, Attar-Levy D *et al.* Binding of antipsychotic drugs to cortical 5-HT2A receptors: a PET study of chlorpromazine, clozapine, and amisulpride in schizophrenic patients. *Am J Psychiatry* 1998; **155**: 505–508.

134. Martinot JL, Paillere-Martinot ML, Poirier MF *et al.* In vivo characteristics of dopamine D2 receptor occupancy by amisulpride in schizophrenia. *Psychopharmacology (Berl)* 1996; **124**: 154–158.

135. Puech A, Fleurot O, Rein W. Amisulpride, and atypical antipsychotic, in the treatment of acute episodes of schizophrenia: a dose-ranging study vs haloperidol. The Amisulpride Study Group. *Acta Psychiatr Scand* 1998; **98**: 65–72.

136. Moller HJ, Boyer P, Fleurot O, Rein W. Improvement of acute exacerbations of schizophrenia with amisulpride: a comparison with haloperidol. PROD-ASLP study group. *Psychopharmacology (Berl)* 1997; **132**: 396–401.

137. Goldstein JM. Pre-clinical pharmacology of new atypical antipsychotics in late stage development. *Exp Opin Invest Drugs* 1995; **4**: 291–298.

138. Moore NA, Calligaro DO, Wong DT *et al.* The pharmacology of olanzapine and other new antipsychotic agents. *Curr Opin Invest Drugs* 1993; **2**: 281–293.

139. Daniel DG, Zimbroff DL, Potkin SG *et al.* Ziprasidone 80 mg/day and 160 mg/day in the acute exacerbation of schizophrenia and

schizoaffective disorder: a 6-week placebo-controlled trial. Ziprasidone Study Group. *Neuropsychopharmacology* 1999; **20**: 491–505.

140. Goff DC, Posever T, Herz L *et al.* An exploratory haloperidol-controlled dose-finding study of ziprasidone in hospitalized patients with schizophrenia or schizoaffective disorder. *J Clin Psychopharmacol* 1998; **18**: 296–304.

141. Ackenheil M. The biochemical effect profile of zotepine in comparison with other neuroleptics. *Fortschr Neurol Psychiatr* 1991; **59**: 2–9.

142. Barnas C, Stuppack CH, Miller C *et al.* Zotepine in the treatment of schizophrenic patients with prevailingly negative symptoms. A double-blind trial vs haloperidol. *Int Clin Psychopharmacol* 1992; **7**: 23–27.

143. Petit M, Raniwalla J, Tweed J *et al.* A comparison of an atypical and typical antipsychotic, zotepine versus haloperidol in patients with acute exacerbation of schizophrenia: a parallel-group double-blind trial. *Psychopharmacol Bull* 1996; **32**: 81–87.

144. Harada T, Otsuki S. Antimanic effect of zotepine. *Clin Ther* 1986; **8**: 406–414.

145. Hori M, Suzuki T, Sasaki M *et al.* Convulsive seizures in schizophrenic patients induced by zotepine administration. *Jpn J Psychiatry Neurol* 1992; **46**: 161–167.

146. Marder SR, Meibach RC. Risperidone in the treatment of schizophrenia. *Am J Psychiatry* 1994; **151**: 825–835.

147. Song F. Risperidone in the treatment of schizophrenia: a meta-analysis of randomized controlled trials. *J Psychopharmacol* 1997; **11**: 65–71.

148. Freeman HL. Amisulpride compared with standard neuroleptics in acute exacerbations of schizophrenia: three efficacy studies. *Int Clin Psychopharmacol* 1997; **12(suppl 2)**: S11–S117.

149. Stacy M, Jankovic J. Tardive dyskinesia. *Curr Opin Neurol Neurosurg* 1991; **4**: 343–349.

150. Naumann R, Felber W, Heilemann H, Reuster T. Olanzapine-induced agranulocytosis. *Lancet* 1999; **354**: 566.

151. Stanton JM. Weight gain associated with neuroleptic medication: a review. *Schizophr Bull* 1995; **21**: 463–472.

152. Loebel AD, Lieberman JA, Alvir JM *et al.* Duration of psychosis and outcome in first-

episode schizophrenia. *Am J Psychiatry* 1992; **149**: 1183–1188.

153. Crow TJ, Macmillan JF, Johnson AL, Johnstone EC. A randomised controlled trial of prophylactic neuroleptic treatment. *Br J Psychiatry* 1986; **148**: 120–127.

154. Remington G, Kapur S, Zipursky RB. Pharmacotherapy of first-episode schizophrenia. *Br J Psychiatry Suppl* 1998; **172**: 66–70.

155. Lieberman J, Jody D, Geisler S *et al.* Time course and biologic correlates of treatment response in first-episode schizophrenia. *Arch Gen Psychiatry* 1993; **50**: 369–376.

156. Zhang-Wong J, Zipursky RB, Beiser M, Bean G. Optimal haloperidol dosage in first-episode psychosis. *Can J Psychiatry* 1999; **44**: 164–167.

157. Sanger TM, Lieberman JA, Tohen M *et al.* Olanzapine versus haloperidol treatment in first-episode psychosis. *Am J Psychiatry* 1999; **156**: 79–87.

158. Tran PV, Hamilton SH, Kuntz AJ *et al.* Double-blind comparison of olanzapine versus risperidone in the treatment of schizophrenia and other psychotic disorders. *J Clin Psychopharmacol* 1997; **17**: 407–418.

159. The drug treatment of patients with schizophrenia. *Drug Ther Bull* 1995; **33**: 81–86.

160. Wiersma D, Nienhuis FJ, Slooff CJ, Giel R. Natural course of schizophrenic disorders: a 15-year followup of a Dutch incidence cohort. *Schizophr Bull* 1998; **24**: 75–85.

161. Bollini P, Pampallona S, Orza MJ *et al.* Antipsychotic drugs: is more worse? A meta-analysis of the published randomized control trials. *Psychol Med* 1994; **24**: 307–316.

162. Gur RE, Pearlson G. Neuroimaging in schizophrenia research. *Schizophr Bull* 1993; **19**: 337–353.

163. Nyberg S, Eriksson B, Oxenstierna G *et al.* Suggested minimal effective dose of risperidone based on PET-measured D2 and 5-HT2A receptor occupancy in schizophrenic patients. *Am J Psychiatry* 1999; **156**: 869–875.

164. Kapur S, Zipursky RB, Remington G *et al.* 5-HT2 and D2 receptor occupancy of olanzapine in schizophrenia: a PET investigation. *Am J Psychiatry* 1998; **155**: 921–928.

165. Lemmens P, Brecher M, Van Baelen B. A

combined analysis of double-blind studies with risperidone vs placebo and other antipsychotic agents: factors associated with extrapyramidal symptoms. *Acta Psychiatr Scand* 1999; **99**: 160–170.

166. Conley RR, Tamminga CA, Kelly DL, Richardson CM. Treatment-resistant schizophrenic patients respond to clozapine after olanzapine non-response. *Biol Psychiatry* 1999; **46**: 73–77.

167. Robinson D, Woerner MG, Alvir JM *et al.* Predictors of relapse following response from a first episode of schizophrenia or schizoaffective disorder. *Arch Gen Psychiatry* 1999; **56**: 241–247.

168. Ohmori T, Ito K, Abekawa T, Koyama T. Psychotic relapse and maintenance therapy in paranoid schizophrenia: a 15 year follow up. *Eur Arch Psychiatry Clin Neurosci* 1999; **249**: 73–78.

169. Gaebel W. Is intermittent, early intervention medication an alternative for neuroleptic maintenance treatment? *Int Clin Psychopharmacol* 1995; **9(suppl 5)**: 11–16.

170. Tran PV, Dellva MA, Tollefson GD *et al.* Oral olanzapine versus oral haloperidol in the maintenance treatment of schizophrenia and related psychoses. *Br J Psychiatry* 1998; **172**: 499–505.

171. Beasley CM, Dellva MA, Tamura RN *et al.* Randomised double-blind comparison of the incidence of tardive dyskinesia in patients with schizophrenia during long-term treatment with olanzapine or haloperidol. *Br J Psychiatry* 1999; **174**: 23–30.

172. Moller HJ, Gagiano CA, Addington DE *et al.* Long-term treatment of chronic schizophrenia with risperidone: an open-label, multicenter study of 386 patients. *Int Clin Psychopharmacol* 1998; **13**: 99–106.

173. Speller JC, Barnes TR, Curson DA *et al.* One-year, low-dose neuroleptic study of in-patients with chronic schizophrenia characterised by persistent negative symptoms. Amisulpride v haloperidol. *Br J Psychiatry* 1997; **171**: 564–568.

174. Gerlach J. Depot neuroleptics in relapse prevention: advantages and disadvantages. *Int Clin Psychopharmacol* 1995; **9(suppl 5)**: 17–20.

175. Davis JM, Metalon L, Watanabe MD, Blake L. Depot antipsychotic drugs. Place in therapy. *Drugs* 1994; **47**: 741–773.

176. Kane J, Honigfeld G, Singer J, Meltzer H. Clozapine for the treatment-resistant schizophrenic. A double-blind comparison with chlorpromazine. *Arch Gen Psychiatry* 1988; **45**: 789–796.

177. Lieberman JA, Safferman AZ, Pollack S *et al*. Clinical effects of clozapine in chronic schizophrenia: response to treatment and predictors of outcome. *Am J Psychiatry* 1994; **151**: 1744–1752.

178. Kane JM. Clinical efficacy of clozapine in treatment-refractory schizophrenia: an overview. *Br J Psychiatry Suppl* 1992; **17**: 41–45.

179. Breier AF, Malhotra AK, Su TP *et al*. Clozapine and risperidone in chronic schizophrenia: effects on symptoms, parkinsonian side effects, and neuroendocrine response. *Am J Psychiatry* 1999; **156**: 294–298.

180. Bondolfi G, Dufour H, Patris M *et al*. Risperidone versus clozapine in treatment-resistant chronic schizophrenia: a randomized double-blind study. The Risperidone Study Group. *Am J Psychiatry* 1998; **155**: 499–504.

181. Lindenmayer JP, Iskander A, Park M *et al*. Clinical and neurocognitive effects of clozapine and risperidone in treatment-refractory schizophrenic patients: a prospective study. *J Clin Psychiatry* 1998; **59**: 521–527.

182. Martin J, Gomez JC, Garcia-Bernardo E *et al*. Olanzapine in treatment-refractory schizophrenia: results of an open-label study. The Spanish Group for the Study of Olanzapine in Treatment-Refractory Schizophrenia. *J Clin Psychiatry* 1997; **58**: 479–483.

183. Breier A, Hamilton SH. Comparative efficacy of olanzapine and haloperidol for patients with treatment-resistant schizophrenia. *Biol Psychiatry* 1999; **45**: 403–411.

184. Conley RR, Tamminga CA, Bartko JJ *et al*. Olanzapine compared with chlorpromazine in treatment-resistant schizophrenia. *Am J Psychiatry* 1998; **155**: 914–920.

185. Henderson DC, Goff DC. Risperidone as an adjunct to clozapine therapy in chronic schizophrenics. *J Clin Psychiatry* 1996; **57**: 395–397.

186. Shiloh R, Zemishlany Z, Aizenberg D *et al*. Sulpiride augmentation in people with schizophrenia partially responsive to clozapine. A double-blind, placebo-controlled study. *Br J Psychiatry* 1997; **171**: 569–573.

187. Barnes TR, McEvedy CJ, Nelson HE. Management of treatment resistant schizophrenia unresponsive to clozapine. *Br J Psychiatry Suppl* 1996; **31**: 31–40.

188. Bebbington PE. The content and context of compliance. *Int Clin Psychopharmacol* 1995; **9(suppl 5)**: 41–50.

189. Fenton WS, Blyler CR, Heinssen RK. Determinants of medication compliance in schizophrenia: empirical and clinical findings. *Schizophr Bull* 1997; **23**: 637–651.

190. Wykes T, Reeder C, Corner J *et al*. The effects of neurocognitive remediation on executive processing in patients with schizophrenia. *Schizophr Bull* 1999; **25**: 291–307.

191. Brenner HD, Hodel B, Roder V, Corrigan P. Treatment of cognitive dysfunctions and behavioral deficits in schizophrenia. *Schizophr Bull* 1992; **18**: 21–26.

192. Spaulding WD, Fleming SK, Reed D *et al*. Cognitive functioning in schizophrenia: implications for psychiatric rehabilitation. *Schizophr Bull* 1999; **25**: 275–289.

193. Haddock G, Tarrier N, Spaulding W *et al*. Individual cognitive-behavior therapy in the treatment of hallucinations and delusions: a review. *Schizophr Res* 1998; **32**: 137–150.

194. Shergill SS, Murray RM, McGuire PK. Auditory hallucinations: a review of psychological treatments. *Schizophr Res* 1998; **32**: 137–150.

195. Kuipers E, Fowler D, Garety P *et al*. London–East Anglia randomised controlled trial of cognitive-behavioural therapy for psychosis. III: Follow-up and economic evaluation at 18 months. *Br J Psychiatry* 1998; **173**: 61–68.

196. Tarrier N, Yusupoff L, Kinney C *et al*. Randomised controlled trial of intensive cognitive behaviour therapy for patients with chronic schizophrenia. *BMJ* 1998; **317**: 303–307.

197. Bebbington P, Kuipers L. The predictive utility of expressed emotion in schizophrenia: an aggregate analysis. *Psychol Med* 1994; **24**: 707–718.

198. Mueser KT, Bellack AS. Psychotherapy for schizophrenia. In: Hirsch SR, Weinberger DR, eds. *Schizophrenia*. Oxford: Blackwell Science, 1995, 626–648.

199. Falloon IRH, Brooker C. A critical re-evaluation of social and family interventions in schizophrenia. *Schizophr Monitor* 1992; **2**: 1–4.

200. Nugter A, Dingemans P, Van der Does JW *et al*. Family treatment, expressed emotion and relapse in recent onset schizophrenia. *Psychiatry Res* 1997; **72**: 23–31.

201. Schooler NR, Keith SJ, Severe JB *et al.* Relapse and rehospitalization during maintenance treatment of schizophrenia. The effects of dose reduction and family treatment. *Arch Gen Psychiatry* 1997; **54**: 453–463.

202. Szmukler GI, Herrman H, Colusa S *et al.* A controlled trial of a counselling intervention for caregivers of relatives with schizophrenia. *Soc Psychiatry Psychiatr Epidemiol* 1996; **31**: 149–155.

203. McFarlane WR, Dushay RA, Stastny P *et al.* A comparison of two levels of family-aided assertive community treatment. *Psychiatr Serv* 1996; **47**: 744–750.

204. McFarlane WR, Lukens E, Link B *et al.* Multiple-family groups and psychoeducation in the treatment of schizophrenia. *Arch Gen Psychiatry* 1995; **52**: 679–687.

205. Goldstein MJ. Psychoeducational and family therapy in relapse prevention. *Acta Psychiatr Scand Suppl* 1994; **382**: 54–57.

206. Merinder LB, Viuff AG, Laugesen HD *et al.* Patient and relative education in community psychiatry: a randomized controlled trial regarding its effectiveness. *Soc Psychiatry Psychiatr Epidemiol* 1999; **34**: 287–294.

207. Wirshing WC, Marder SR, Eckman T *et al.* Acquisition and retention of skills training methods in chronic schizophrenic outpatients. *Psychopharmacol Bull* 1992; **28**: 241–245.

208. Kendell RE, Chalmers JC, Platz C. Epidemiology of puerperal psychoses. *Br J Psychiatry* 1987; **150**: 662–673.

209. Kumar R, Marks M, Platz C, Yoshida K. Clinical survey of a psychiatric mother and baby unit: characteristics of 100 consecutive admissions. *J Affect Disord* 1995; **33**: 11–22.

210. Spielvogel A, Wile J. Treatment and outcomes of psychotic patients during pregnancy and childbirth. *Birth* 1992; **19**: 131–137.

211. Altshuler LL, Szuba MP. Course of psychiatric disorders in pregnancy. Dilemmas in pharmacologic management. *Neurol Clin* 1994; **12**: 613–635.

212. Cannon TD, Mednick SA, Parnas J *et al.* Developmental brain abnormalities in the offspring of schizophrenic mothers. I. Contributions of genetic and perinatal factors. *Arch Gen Psychiatry* 1993; **50**: 551–564.

213. Siris SG. Diagnosis of secondary depression

in schizophrenia: implications for DSM-IV. *Schizophr Bull* 1991; **17**: 75–98.

214. Johnson DAW. Studies of depressive symptoms in schizophrenia. *Br J Psychiatry* 1981; **139**: 89–101.

215. Hafner H, Loffler W, Maurer K, Hambrecht M, van der Heiden W. Depression, negative symptoms, social decline in the early course of schizophrenia. *Acta Psychiatr Scand* 1999; **100**: 105–118.

216. Hirsch SR, Jolley AG, Barnes TR *et al.* Dysphoric and depressive symptoms in chronic schizophrenia. *Schizophr Res* 1989; **2**: 259–264.

217. Barnes TR, Curson DA, Liddle PF, Patel M. The nature and prevalence of depression in chronic schizophrenic in-patients. *Br J Psychiatry* 1989; **154**: 486–491.

218. Wiersma D, Nienhuis FJ, Slooff CJ, Giel R. Natural course of schizophrenic disorders: a 15-year followup of a Dutch incidence cohort. *Schizophr Bull* 1998; **24**: 75–85.

219. Heila H, Isometsa ET, Henriksson MM *et al.* Suicide and schizophrenia: a nationwide psychological autopsy study on age- and sex-specific clinical characteristics of 92

suicide victims with schizophrenia. *Am J Psychiatry* 1997; **154**: 1235–1242.

220. Mauri MC, Bitetto A, Fabiano L *et al.* Depressive symptoms and schizophrenic relapses: the effect of four neuroleptic drugs. *Prog Neuropsychopharmacol Biol Psychiatry* 1999; **23**: 43–54.

221. Dufresne RL, Valentino D, Kass DJ. Thioridazine improves affective symptoms in schizophrenic patients. *Psychopharmacol Bull* 1993; **29**: 249–255.

222. Krakowski M, Czobor P, Volavka J. Effect of neuroleptic treatment on depressive symptoms in acute schizophrenic episodes. *Psychiatry Res* 1997; **71**: 19–26.

223. Levinson DF, Umapathy C, Musthaq M. Treatment of schizoaffective disorder and schizophrenia with mood symptoms. *Am J Psychiatry* 1999; **156**: 1138–1148.

224. Marder SR, Davis JM, Chouinard G. The effects of risperidone on the five dimensions of schizophrenia derived by factor analysis: combined results of the North American trials. *J Clin Psychiatry* 1997; **58**: 538–546.

225. Tollefson GD, Sanger TM. Anxious–depressive symptoms in schizophrenia: a new treatment target for

pharmacotherapy? *Schizophr Res* 1999; **35(suppl)**: S13–S21.

226. Delcker A, Schoon ML, Oczkowski B, Gaertner HJ. Amisulpride versus haloperidol in treatment of schizophrenic patients: results of a double-blind study. *Pharmacopsychiatry* 1990; **23**: 125–130.

227. Daniel DG, Zimbroff DL, Potkin SG *et al.* Ziprasidone 80 mg/day and 160 mg/day in the acute exacerbation of schizophrenia and schizoaffective disorder: a 6-week placebo-controlled trial. Ziprasidone Study Group. *Neuropsychopharmacology* 1999; **20**: 491–505.

228. Meltzer HY, Okayli G. Reduction of suicidality during clozapine treatment of neuroleptic-resistant schizophrenia: impact on risk–benefit assessment. *Am J Psychiatry* 1995; **152**: 183–190.

229. Siris SG, van Kammen DP, Docherty JP. Use of antidepressant drugs in schizophrenia. *Arch Gen Psychiatry* 1978; **35**: 1368–1377.

230. Siris SG, Bermanzohn PC, Mason SE, Shuwall MA. Maintenance imipramine therapy for secondary depression in schizophrenia. A controlled trial. *Arch Gen Psychiatry* 1994; **51**: 109–115.

231. Dose M, Hellweg R, Yassouridis A *et al.* Combined treatment of schizophrenic psychoses with haloperidol and valproate. *Pharmacopsychiatry* 1998; **31**: 122–125.

232. Hafner H, Boker W. *Crimes of Violence by Mentally Abnormal Offenders.* Cambridge: Cambridge University Press, 1973.

233. Rasanen P, Tiihonen J, Isohanni M *et al.* Schizophrenia, alcohol abuse, and violent behavior: a 26-year followup study of an unselected birth cohort. *Schizophr Bull* 1998; **24**: 437–441.

234. Wessely S. The Camberwell Study of Crime and Schizophrenia. *Soc Psychiatry Psychiatr Epidemiol* 1998; **33(suppl 1)**: S24–S28.

235. Taylor PJ. Schizophrenia and the risk of violence. In: Hirsch SR, Weinberger DR, eds. *Schizophrenia.* Oxford: Blackwell Science, 1995, 163–183.

236. Taylor PJ, Parrott JM. Elderly offenders. A study of age-related factors among custodially remanded prisoners. *Br J Psychiatry* 1988; **152**: 340–346.

237. Taylor PJ, Leese M, Williams D *et al.* Mental disorder and violence. A special (high security) hospital study. *Br J Psychiatry* 1998; **172**: 218–226.

238. Swartz MS, Swanson JW, Hiday VA *et al.*
     Taking the wrong drugs: the role of
     substance abuse and medication
     noncompliance in violence among severely
     mentally ill individuals. *Soc Psychiatry
     Psychiatr Epidemiol* 1998; **33(suppl 1)**:
     S75–S80.

239. Nolan KA, Volavka J, Mohr P, Czobor P.
     Psychopathy and violent behavior among
     patients with schizophrenia or
     schizoaffective disorder. *Psychiatr Serv*
     1999; **50**: 787–792.

240. Modestin J. Criminal and violent behavior
     in schizophrenic patients: an overview.
     Psychiatry Clin Neurosci 1998; **52**: 547–554.

241. Chiswick D. Forensic Psychiatry. In:
     Kendell RE, Zealley AK, eds. *Companion to
     Psychiatric Studies* 5th ed. Edinburgh:
     Churchill-Livingstone, 1993, 793–816.

242. Estroff SE, Swanson JW, Lachicotte WS *et
     al.* Risk reconsidered: targets of violence in
     the social networks of people with serious
     psychiatric disorders. *Soc Psychiatry
     Psychiatr Epidemiol* 1998; **33(suppl 1)**:
     S95–S101.

243. *British National Formulary.* London: British
     Medical Association and Royal
     Pharmaceutical Society of Great Britain,
     1998, 219.

244. Volavka J. The effects of clozapine on
     aggression and substance abuse in
     schizophrenic patients. *J Clin Psychiatry*
     1999; **60(suppl 12)**: 43–46.

245. Davies LM, Drummond MF. Economics
     and schizophrenia: the real cost. *Br J
     Psychiatry Suppl* 1994; 18–21.

246. Evers SM, Ament AJ. Costs of
     schizophrenia in The Netherlands.
     Schizophr Bull 1995; **21**: 141–153.

247. Rouillon F, Dansette GY, Le Floch C.
     Therapeutic management of schizophrenic
     patients and its cost. *Encephale* 1994; **20**:
     303–309.

248. Davies LM, Drummond MF. Assessment
     of costs and benefits of drug therapy for
     treatment-resistant schizophrenia in the
     United Kingdom. *Br J Psychiatry* 1993;
     162: 38–42.

249. Maynard A, Bloor K. Building castles on
     sands or quicksands? The strengths and
     weaknesses of economic evaluation in
     pharmaceuticals. *Br J Psychiatry Suppl*
     1998; **36**: 12–18.

250. Udvarhelyi IS, Colditz GA, Rai A, Epstein
     AM. Cost-effectiveness and costs–benefit
     analyses in the medical literature. Are the
     methods being used correctly? *Ann Intern
     Med* 1992; **116**: 238–244.

251. Adams ME, McCall NT, Gray DT *et al.* Economic analysis in randomized control trials. *Med Care* 1992; **30:** 231–243.

252. Meltzer HY, Cola P, Way L *et al.* Cost effectiveness of clozapine in neuroleptic-resistant schizophrenia. *Am J Psychiatry* 1993; **150:** 1630–1638.

253. Foster RH, Goa KL. Risperidone. A pharmacoeconomic review of its use in schizophrenia. *Pharmacoeconomics* 1998; **14:** 97–133.

254. Revicki DA. Pharmacoeconomic studies of atypical antipsychotic drugs for the treatment of schizophrenia. *Schizophr Res* 1999; **35(suppl):** S101–S109.

255. Kind P, Sorenson J. The costs of depression. *Int Clin Psychopharmacol* 1993; **7:** 191–195.

256. Meltzer H, Gill B, Petticrew M, Hinds K. Prevalence of psychiatric disorders. In: *The Prevalence of Psychiatric Morbidity Among Adults Living in Private Households.* London: Her Majesty's Stationery Office: 1995, 66–94.

257. McGuire TG. Measuring the economic costs of schizophrenia. *Schizophr Bull* 1991; **17:** 375–388.

Index